Combination Therapy
in Hypertension

Combination Therapy in Hypertension

Joel M Neutel
Department of Medicine,
University of California in Irvine,
Irvine, California, USA

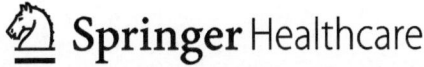

Published by Springer Healthcare Ltd, 236 Gray's Inn Road, London WC1X 8HB, UK

www.springerhealthcare.com

© 2011 Springer Healthcare, a part of Springer Science+Business Media

ISBN 978-1-908517-25-8

British Library Cataloguing-in-Publication Data.
A catalogue record for this book is available from the British Library.

Although every effort has been made to ensure that drug doses and other information are presented accurately in this publication, the ultimate responsibility rests with the prescribing physician. Neither the publisher nor the authors can be held responsible for errors or for any consequences arising from the use of the information contained herein. Any product mentioned in this publication should be used in accordance with the prescribing information prepared by the manufacturers. No claims or endorsements are made for any drug or compound at present under clinical investigation.

Commissioning editor: Dinah Alam
Project editor: Alison Whitehouse
Designer: Joe Harvey
Production: Marina Maher
Printed in xxx by xxx

Contents

Contents

Author biography

Joel M Neutel is Associate Professor of Medicine in the Department of Medicine at the University of California in Irvine. He is also Medical Director of Clinical Pharmacology at Orange County Research Center in Tustin. He began his medical training at the University of Witwatersrand in Johannesburg, South Africa, completing his residencies at Johannesburg Hospital, J.G. Strydom Hospital in Johannesburg, VA Medical Center, and the University of California. He is a member of and a specialist in clinical hypertension for the American Society of Hypertension and is a member of the Society of Geriatric Cardiology. He has published many papers and book chapters, and serves on the editorial boards of *Cardiovascular Drugs and Therapy* and *The Journal of Clinical Hypertension,* as well as being a reviewer for *Hypertension, Blood Pressure Monitoring, Journal of Human Hypertension, American Journal of Hypertension,* and *American Heart Journal.*

Chapter 1

State of hypertension control

Almost one billion individuals worldwide are currently estimated to be affected by hypertension, or high blood pressure, with this figure predicted to rise to over 1.5 billion by 2025 [1]. Significantly, approximately one-half of this affected population is unaware of the condition [2], and, of those who are aware, more than half have not been treated [3].

Hypertension is a major, and growing, global public health problem, contributing an enormous disease burden (hypertension is estimated to cause 4.5% of current global disease burden [4]), premature morbidity and mortality [5–7]. Elevated blood pressure is a massive health problem in almost every country worldwide [8]: it is prevalent in many developing countries (though the lack of blood pressure data in developing countries is substantial [9]), as well as in the developed world, where more than one in five adults [10] has been estimated to have hypertension. Nearly two-thirds of individuals with hypertension live in low- and middle-income countries, which means that it comprises a massive economic burden [11].

Classification of blood pressure for adults has recently changed. The current recommendation by the US Joint National Committee on Prevention, Detection, Evaluation, and Treatment of High Blood Pressure [12] and the World Health Organization for adequate control of hypertension (i.e. normal blood pressure) is 130/85 mmHg for uncomplicated hypertension, which is 10/5 mmHg lower than the previous limit of 140/90 mmHg (Figure 1.1). In patients with underlying coronary artery disease, the recommended target blood pressure is 120/80 mmHg, and in patients with diabetic nephropathy, 125/75 mmHg is associated with greater renoprotection. Although new, lower target blood pressure levels have been recommended, the blood pressure that is universally accepted to represent adequate control of hypertension in medical practice continues to be 140/90 mmHg for all patients, apart from those with diabetes or renal disease, in whom 130/80 mmHg is the target level.

J. M. Neutel, *Combination Therapy in Hypertension*,
DOI: 10.1007/978-1-908517-28-9_1, © Springer Healthcare 2011

Classification of blood pressure for adults			
	Blood pressure (mmHg)		
Category	**Systolic**		**Diastolic**
Optimal	<120	and	<80
Normal	<130	and	<85
Prehypertension	120–139	or	80–89
Hypertension			
Stage 1	140–159	or	90–99
Stage 2	≥160	or	≥100

Figure 1.1 Classification of blood pressure for adults. Reproduced with permission from The Seventh Report of the Joint National Committee on Prevention, Detection, Evaluation, and Treatment of High Blood Pressure. Bethesda, MD: US Department of Health and Human Services. August 2004.

Hypertension and cardiovascular risk

Hypertension is a well-documented risk factor for cardiovascular disease [13] and is a major contributor to worldwide cardiovascular mortality [14]. Elevated blood pressure is one of the primary risk factors for heart disease and stroke, which are the leading causes of death worldwide. Factors such as increasing longevity and obesity contribute to the prevalence of hypertension and the associated cardiovascular risk [15]. The incidence of hypertension in obese individuals is five times that in individuals of normal weight, and the risk of cardiovascular disease is considerably greater in the obese population compared with the normal weight population [16]. Treated hypertensive patients who smoke have a worse cardiovascular risk profile than treated hypertensive patients who do not smoke, which indicates that the negative effect of smoking may outweigh the benefit of blood pressure control [17].

Blood pressure-induced cardiovascular risk rises continuously across the whole blood pressure range [4]. Systolic blood pressure is a better predictor of pending cardiovascular disease than diastolic blood pressure; furthermore, high systolic blood pressure is more difficult to control than high diastolic blood pressure. Cardiovascular mortality risk has been shown to be doubled for each 20 mmHg increase in systolic blood pressure (or, approximately equivalently, 10 mmHg diastolic blood pressure) in subjects aged from 40 to 69 years (Figure 1.2) [18].

Target blood pressure

Recent epidemiological analyses have changed the way that hypertension is viewed: cardiovascular risk has been found to be elevated at levels of blood pressure previously believed to be normal and not imparting additional risk

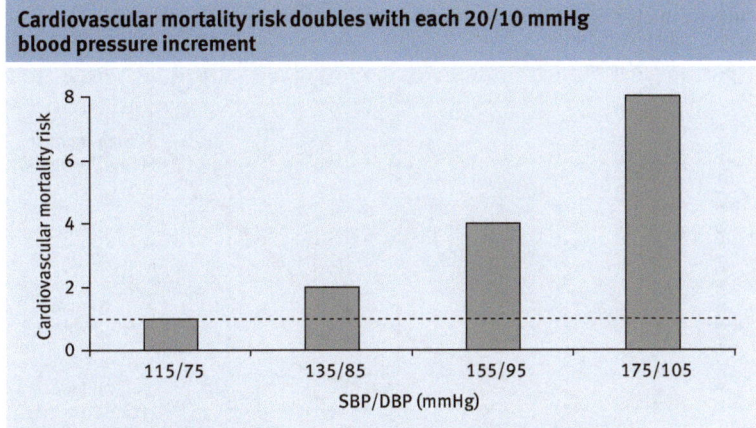

Figure 1.2 Cardiovascular mortality risk doubles with each 20/10 mmHg blood pressure increment. Individuals aged 40–69 years, starting at BP 115/75 mmHg. SBP, systolic blood pressure; DBP, diastolic blood pressure.

[19]. For example, the impact of high-normal blood pressure (systolic/diastolic blood pressure of 130–139/85–89 mmHg, which was previously regarded as normal) on cardiovascular disease risk is shown in Figure 1.3 [20]. These findings prompted the lowering of the blood pressure limit that is regarded as representing adequate control of hypertension (see above).

Epidemiological data have established a continuous relationship between blood pressure and cardiovascular risk that extends down to systolic/diastolic blood pressure levels as low as 115/75 mmHg, which emphasizes the lack of a critical threshold value that defines 'high' blood pressure [21]. Consideration of the continuous relationship between blood pressure and cardiovascular risk has led to the introduction of a new category of hypertension, called pre-hypertension, which includes individuals with a systolic blood pressure between 120 and 139 mmHg and/or a diastolic blood pressure between 80 and 89 mmHg [12,21,22]. To put this category into perspective, a total of 70 million individuals in the USA (approximately 30% of the population) has been estimated to have pre-hypertension [21]. The risk of cardiovascular disease in this large population is not uniform: it increases with rising concomitant burden of other cardiovascular risk factors [21].

Levels of blood pressure control around the world

The capacity for and capability in management of hypertension vary greatly between different countries. The worldwide picture, from the US National

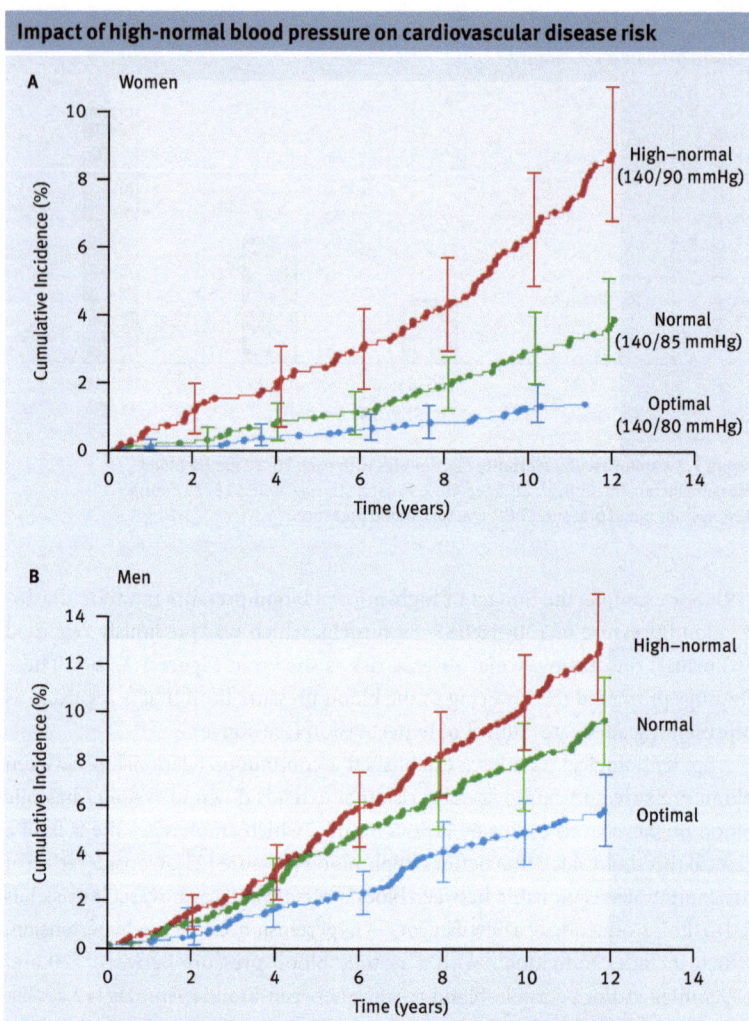

Figure 1.3 Impact of high-normal blood pressure (BP) on cardiovascular disease risk.
Optimal BP: <120/80 mmHg; normal BP: 120–129/80–84 mmHg; high-normal:
130–139/85–89 mmHg. Reproduced with permission from Vasan RS, Larson MG,
Leip EP, et al. Impact of high-normal blood pressure on the risk of cardiovascular
disease. N Engl J Med 2001; 345(18):1291–7.

Health and Nutritional Examination Survey (Figure 1.4) and the World Health
Organization, shows that less than 30% of individuals who are diagnosed with
the condition are adequately controlled according to currently accepted blood

pressure goals [4,26]. Furthermore, although many different antihypertensive agents are available, the majority of treated hypertensives fail to achieve blood pressure control to less than 140/90 mmHg [27].

Published evidence of low rates of blood pressure control is available from several different European countries. For example, a great improvement in the efficacy of hypertension management has been reported to have taken place in England between 1994 and 2003, with more awareness, treatment, and control; however, in 2003, the majority of adults with hypertension in England had blood pressure levels above the currently recommended targets [28]. Control rates (<140 mmHg systolic and <90 mmHg diastolic) among hypertensive men and women in 2003 were 21.5% and 22.8%, respectively [28].

Further evidence of inadequately controlled hypertension in treated patients is provided by a cross-sectional study conducted to assess the prevalence, level of awareness, treatment, and control of hypertension in Greece [29]. Data from a total of 11 540 individuals (0.1% of the Greek population) were analyzed: 31% of these individuals had hypertension, 40% of whom were unaware that they had hypertension, and 12% of whom were aware but not treated. In total, 51% of individuals with hypertension were treated: 67% of the treated individuals were not controlled, and 33% were treated and controlled [29].

Poor rates of blood pressure control have also been reported in a multi-center, cross-sectional study conducted in Spain [30]. A total of 73% of the 7343 participants in the study had hypertension. Among the individuals with hypertension, 29% had blood pressure on therapeutic objective and, of the total population, 36% had blood pressure under control [30]. Poor control of hypertension was reported to be one of the main factors related to stroke mortality rates after controlling for age, gender, obesity, diabetes, and urban setting [30].

Hypertension awareness, treatment and control in people who have hypertension							
Category	NHANES II	NHANES III (phase 1)	(phase 2)				
	1976–1980	1988–1991	1991–1994	1999–2000	2001–2002	2003–2004	2005–2006
Aware (%)	51.0	73.0	68.4	68.7	70.7	75.7	78.0
Treated (%)	31.0	55.0	53.6	58.2	60.1	65.1	68.0
Controlled* (%)	10.0	29.0	27.6	29.2	32.5	36.8	43.5

Figure 1.4 Hypertension awareness, treatment and control in people who have hypertension.
*Controlled blood pressure = systolic blood pressure <140 mmHg and diastolic blood pressure <90 mmHg. Data from Neutel [23], Ong et al. [24], and Ostchega et al. [25].

Awareness of hypertension has improved greatly in the last 20 years in the Czech Republic and the prevalence of this condition has markedly decreased [31]. Control of hypertension has also improved significantly over this period; however, control rates of only 18% were reported in 2000/2001 [31].

Over 50% of adults have uncontrolled hypertension in the Republic of Georgia [32]. Similarly poor rates of control have been reported in the USA and Canada: only around one-third [33] (37%) of individuals with hypertension in the USA currently have their blood pressure adequately controlled, compared with less than 15% of those in Canada [34,35].

Effect of blood pressure control on cardiovascular and cerebrovascular risk

Many factors contribute to poor control of blood pressure; the most important are shown in Figure 1.5 [26]. Poor control places the hypertensive patient at significant risk for the development of cardiovascular disease. Indeed, the recognition of hypertension as a disease process came from epidemiological studies that showed that increased blood pressure was associated with an increased incidence of cardiovascular events [36]. As a result, the primary goal in the management of hypertension has always been to reduce the incidence of cardiovascular events in hypertensive patients to the levels seen in normotensive subjects [23,26,36]. Treatment of hypertension to produce effective blood pressure control has been shown to dramatically reduce the incidence of stroke, but reductions in the incidence of coronary artery disease have been very disappointing [26,37–40]. For example, the incidence of coronary artery disease is higher in treated hypertensive patients than in matched normal controls, despite similar blood pressure levels [41].

Figure 1.6 shows the disparity between the effect of antihypertensive therapy on cerebrovascular disease and that on coronary artery disease [42]. The reasons for the poor results in coronary artery disease are probably numerous, but the two primary reasons are:

Factors that contribute to poor blood pressure control

- Lack of patient compliance with antihypertensive treatment
  Most important reason

- Reluctance of physicians to titrate antihypertensive medication
  (usually for a good reason)

- Adequate blood pressure control with monotherapy is very difficult or impossible to achieve in the majority of patients

Figure 1.5 Factors that contribute to poor blood pressure control.

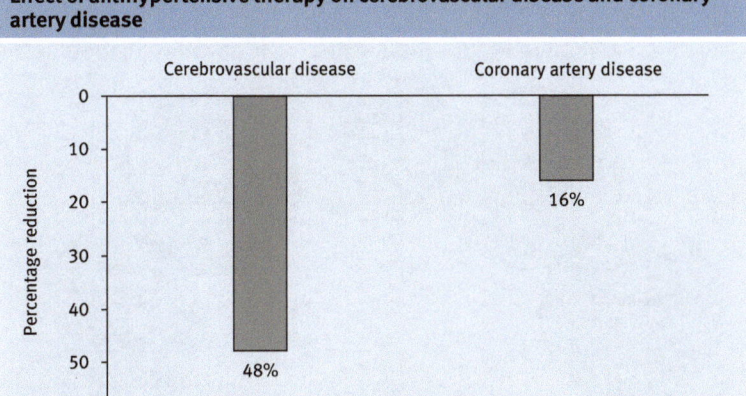

Figure 1.6 Effect of antihypertensive therapy on cerebrovascular disease and coronary artery disease. Reproduced with permission from MacMahon SW, Cutler JA, Furberg CD, Payne GH. The effects of drug treatment for hypertension on morbidity and mortality from cardiovascular disease: a review of randomized controlled trials. Progr Cardiovasc Dis 1986; 29(3 Suppl 1):99–118.

1. Hypertension is a complex inherited syndrome of cardiovascular risk factors, all of which are genetically linked and all of which contribute to the development of cardiovascular disease (Figure 1.7) [43,44]:
   - factors other than blood pressure are associated with the development of coronary artery disease in patients with hypertension [45]
   - in many patients, hypertension is a late manifestation of the disease process
   - all components of the hypertension syndrome must be considered in the treatment of this condition to impact on the incidence of cardiovascular disease in hypertensive patients [46,47].
2. The majority of hypertensive patients are inadequately controlled:
   - inadequately controlled hypertensive patients, even if they are on antihypertensive medication, are at significant risk for coronary artery disease.

Summary

Rates of control of hypertension remain alarmingly low worldwide despite the extensive evidence for decreased rates of cardiovascular, cerebrovascular, and renal events in response to lowering of blood pressure to recommended targets [48,49]. Furthermore, suboptimal rates of control continue even with advances

Factors that contribute to metabolic hypertension syndrome

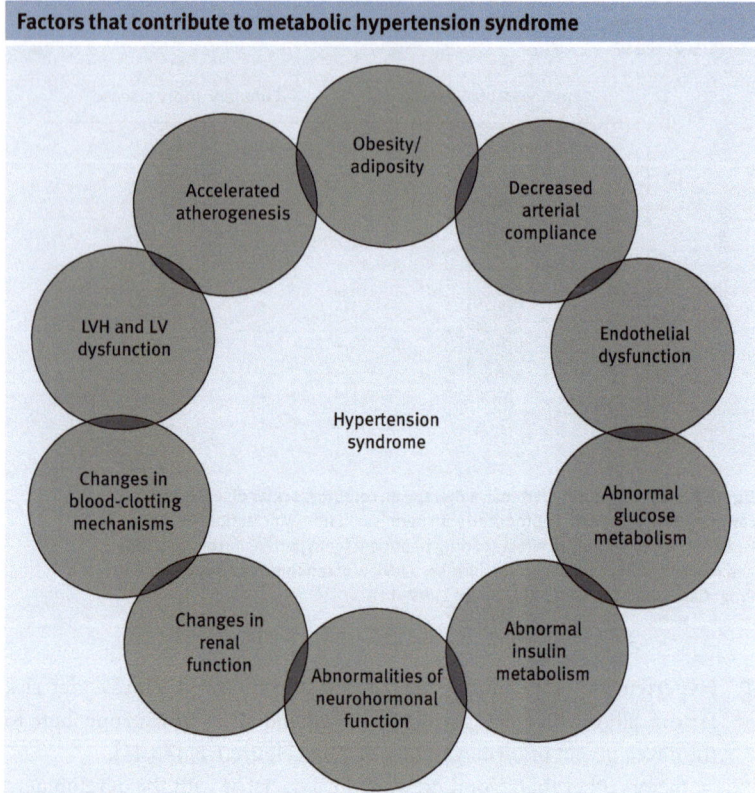

Figure 1.7 Factors that contribute to metabolic hypertension syndrome. LVH, left ventricular hypertrophy.

in the treatment of hypertension [33]. Although administration of antihypertensive therapy has been shown to extend and enhance life, hypertension remains inadequately managed everywhere [15]. Evidently, hypertension is an important public health challenge worldwide [1]. Measures that improve the awareness, prevention, detection, treatment, and control of hypertension are urgently required. Although patient-related factors clearly contribute to poor control of hypertension, physician-related factors, including 'passive' therapeutic inertia [48], and suboptimal adherence to treatment guidelines [50] have been suggested to be at least as responsible. Intensive blood pressure control is a desirable and obtainable goal in patients with hypertension [51]. Hypertension control can be improved in all patient groups, even in healthcare systems with limited resources [32]. This book assesses the use of combination therapy in the treatment of hypertension in the quest to improve rates of control of hypertension.

References

1. Kearney PM, Whelton M, Reynolds K, Muntner P, Whelton PK, He J. Global burden of hypertension: analysis of worldwide data. Lancet 2005; 365(9455):217–23.

2. Chockalingam A. Impact of World Hypertension Day. Can J Cardiol 2007; 23(7):517–19.

3. Chockalingam A. Editorial. News from the World Hypertension League (WHL). A division of the International Society of Hypertension, and in official relations with the World Health Organization. No. 107, June 2006.

4. Whitworth JA; World Health Organization, International Society of Hypertension Writing Group. 2003 World Health Organization (WHO)/International Society of Hypertension (ISH) statement on management of hypertension. J Hypertens 2003; 21(11):1983–92.

5. Ram CV. Hypertension, possible vascular protection and lercanidipine. Expert Rev Cardiovasc Ther 2006; 4(6):783–8.

6. Elliott WJ. Systemic hypertension. Curr Probl Cardiol 2007; 32(4):201–59.

7. Lawes CM, Vander Hoorn S, Law MR, Elliott P, MacMahon S, Rodgers A. Blood pressure and the global burden of disease 2000. Part II: estimates of attributable burden. J Hypertens 2006; 24(3):423–30.

8. Hypertension control. Report of a WHO Expert Committee. Technical Report Series, no. 862. Geneva: WHO, 1996.

9. Lawes CM, Vander Hoorn S, Law MR, Elliott P, MacMahon S, Rodgers A. Blood pressure and the global burden of disease 2000. Part 1: estimates of blood pressure levels. J Hypertens 2006; 24(3):413–22.

10. Vasan RS, Beiser A, Seshadri S, et al. Residual lifetime risk for developing hypertension in middle-aged women and men: The Framingham Heart Study. JAMA 2002; 287(8):1003–10.

11. Chockalingam A, Campbell NR, Fodor JG. Worldwide epidemic of hypertension. Can J Cardiol 2006; 22(7):553–5.

12. The Seventh Report of the Joint National Committee on Prevention, Detection, Evaluation, and Treatment of High Blood Pressure. US Department of Health and Human Services. NIH Publication No. 04-5230. Bethesda, MD: National Institutes of Health, August 2004.

13. Nilsson PM. Optimizing the pharmacologic treatment of hypertension: BP control and target organ protection. Am J Cardiovasc Drugs 2006; 6(5):287–95.

14. Ho PM, Rumsfeld JS. Beyond inpatient and outpatient care: alternative model for hypertension management. BMC Public Health 2006; 6:257.

15. World Health Organization. 2003 Summary: www.who.int/ cardiovascular_diseases/ guidelines/hypertension/en. Last accessed May 2011.

16. Hossain P, Kawar B, El Nahas M. Obesity and diabetes in the developing world – a growing challenge. N Engl J Med 2007; 356(3):213–15.

17. Journath G, Nilsson PM, Petersson U, Paradis BA, Theobald H, Erhardt L. Hypertensive smokers have a worse cardiovascular risk profile than non-smokers in spite of treatment – a national study in Sweden. Blood Press 2005; 14(3):144–50.

18. Lewington S, Clarke R, Qizilbash N, Peto R, Collins R; Prospective Studies Collaboration. Age-specific relevance of usual blood pressure to vascular mortality: a meta-analysis of individual data for one million adults in 61 prospective studies. Lancet 2002; 360(9349):1903–13.

19. Khosla N, Black HR. Expanding the definition of hypertension to incorporate global cardiovascular risk. Curr Hypertens Rep 2006; 8(5):384–90.

20. Vasan RS, Larson MG, Leip EP, et al. Impact of high-normal blood pressure on the risk of cardiovascular disease. N Engl J Med 2001; 345(18):1291–7.

21. Atilla K, Vasan RS. Prehypertension and risk of cardiovascular disease. Expert Rev Cardiovasc Ther 2006; 4(1):111–17.

22. Chobanian AV, Bakris GL, Black HR, et al., National Heart, Lung, and Blood Institute Joint National Committee on Prevention, Detection, Evaluation, and Treatment of High Blood Pressure; National High Blood Pressure Education Program Coordinating Committee. The Seventh Report of the Joint National Committee on Prevention, Detection, Evaluation, and Treatment of High Blood Pressure: the JNC 7 report. JAMA 2003; 289(19):2560–72. Epub 2003 May 14.

23. Neutel JM. Combination therapy and the treatment of hypertension. Cardiology Special Edition 2003; 9(1 of 2):11–15.

24. Ong KL, Cheung BM, Man YB, Lau CP, Lam KS. Prevalence, awareness, treatment, and control of hypertension among United States adults 1999–2004. Hypertension 2007; 49:69–75.

25. Ostchega Y, Sug Yoon S, Hughes J, Louis T, Division of Health and Nutrition Examination Surveys. Control – continued disparities in adults: United States, 2005–2006. NCHS Data Brief, no. 3. Hyattsville, MD: National Center for Health Statistics, January 2008. http://www.cdc.gov/nchs/data/databriefs/db03.pdf. Last accessed May 2011.

26. Neutel JM. The use of combination drug therapy in the treatment of hypertension. Prog Cardiovasc Nurs 2002; 17(2):81–8.

27. Flack JM. Epidemiology and unmet needs in hypertension. J Manag Care Pharm 2007; 13(8 Suppl B):2–8.

28. Primatesta P, Poulter NR. Improvement in hypertension management in England: results from the Health Survey for England 2003. J Hypertens 2006; 24(6):1187–92.

29. Efstratopoulos AD, Voyaki SM, Baltas AA, et al. Prevalence, awareness, treatment and control of hypertension in Hellas, Greece: the Hypertension Study in General Practice in Hellas (HYPERTENSHELL) national study. Am J Hypertens 2006; 19(1):53–60.

30. Redón J, Cea-Calvo L, Lozano JV, et al.; for the PREV-ICTUS study. Differences in blood pressure control and stroke mortality across Spain: the Prevención de Riesgo de Ictus (PREV-ICTUS) study. Hypertension 2007; 49(4):799–805.

31. Cífková R. Arterial hypertension as a public health issue in the Czech Republic. Blood Press Suppl 2005; 2:25–8.

32. Barbakadze VY, Koblianidze LG, Kipshidze NN, Grim CE, Grim CM, Tavill F. The Republic of Georgia High Blood Pressure Control Program. Ethn Dis 2006; 16(2 Suppl 2):S2-61–5.

33. Hajjar I, Kotchen JM, Kotchen TA. Hypertension: trends in prevalence, incidence, and control. Annu Rev Public Health 2006; 27:465–90.

34. Joffres MR, Hamet P, MacLean DR, L'italien GJ, Fodor G. Distribution of blood pressure and hypertension in Canada and the United States. Am J Hypertens 2001; 14(11 Pt 1):1099–105.

35. McLean D, Kingsbury K, Costello JA, Cloutier L, Matheson S; Canadian Hypertension Education Program. 2007 Hypertension Education Program (CHEP) recommendations: management of hypertension by nurses. Can J Cardiovasc Nurs 2007; 17(2):10–16.

36. Neutel JM. Introduction. Am J Hypertens 2001; 14:1S–2S.

37. Samuelsson OG, Wilhelmsen LW, Svärdsudd KF, Pennert KM, Wedel H, Berglund GL. Mortality and morbidity in relation to systolic blood pressure in two populations

with different management of hypertension: the study of men born in 1913 and the multifactorial primary prevention trial. J Hypertens 1987; 5:57–66.

38. Grimm RH Jr, Flack JM, Byington R, Bond G, Brugger S. A comparison of antihypertensive drug effects on the progression of extracranial carotid atherosclerosis. The Multicenter Isradipine Diuretic Atherosclerosis Study (MIDAS). Drugs 1990; 40(Suppl 2):38–43.

39. Moan A, Os I, Hjermann I, Kjeldsen SE. Hypertension therapy and risk of coronary heart disease: how do antihypertensives affect metabolic factors? Cardiology 1995; 86(2):89–93.

40. Gueyffier F, Boissel JP, Boutitie F, et al. Effect of antihypertensive treatment in patients having already suffered from stroke. Gathering the evidence. The INDANA (INdividual Data ANalysis of Antihypertensive intervention trials) Project Collaborators. Stroke 1997; 28(12):2557–62.

41. Havlik RJ, LaCroix AZ, Kleinman JC, Ingram DD, Harris T, Cornoni-Huntley J. Antihypertensive drug therapy and survival by treatment status in a national survey. Hypertension 1989; 13(Suppl):I28–32.

42. MacMahon SW, Cutler JA, Furberg CD, Payne GH. The effects of drug treatment for hypertension on morbidity and mortality from cardiovascular disease: a review of randomized controlled trials. Prog Cardiovasc Dis 1986; 29(3 Suppl 1):99–118.

43. Neutel JM. Hypertension and its management: a problem in need of new treatment strategies. J Renin Angiotensin Aldosterone Syst 2000; 1(Suppl 2):10–13.

44. Weber MA, Smith DH, Neutel JM, Graettinger WF. The therapeutic implications of left ventricular hypertrophy in the hypertensive patient. Am J Ther 1995; 2(12):972–7.

45. Neutel JM, Smith DH, Graettinger WF, Winer RL, Weber MA. Heredity and hypertension: impact on metabolic characteristics. Am Heart J 1992; 124:435–40.

46. Tatti P, Pahor M, Byington RP, et al. Outcome results of the fosinopril versus amlodipine cardiovascular events randomized trial (FACET) in patients with hypertension and NIDDM. Diabetes Care 1998; 21:597–603.

47. Furberg CD, Psaty BM, Pahor M, Alderman MH. Clinical implications of recent findings from the Antihypertensive and Lipid-Lowering Treatment to Prevent Heart Attack Trial (ALLHAT) and other studies of hypertension. Ann Intern Med 2001; 135:1074–8.

48. Collins R, Peto R, MacMahon S, et al. Blood pressure, stroke, and coronary heart disease. Part 2, Short-term reductions in blood pressure: overview of randomised drug trials in their epidemiological context. Lancet 1990; 335:827–38.

49. Ruzicka M, Leenen FH. Moving beyond guidelines: are report cards the answer to high rates of uncontrolled hypertension? Curr Hypertens Rep 2006; 8(4):324–9.

50. Julius S, Cohn JN, Neutel J, et al. Antihypertensive utility of perindopril in a large, general practice-based clinical trial. J Clin Hypertens 2004; 6(1):10–17.

51. Unger T, McInnes GT, Neutel JM, Böhm M. The role of olmesartan medoxomil in the management of hypertension. Drugs 2004; 64(24):2731–9.

Chapter 2

Historical review of combination therapy

Multifactorial approach to the treatment of hypertension

Hypertension is a multi-etiological disease for which a multifactorial treatment approach has been advocated [1]. The multifactorial approach comprises lifestyle modification and/or administration of antihypertensive medications (Figure 2.1).

The main modifiable causes of hypertension are shown in Figure 2.2. Lifestyle modification to address some, or all, of these factors will definitely reduce blood pressure in hypertensive patients; however, it is possible to rely on this type of treatment too long. Non-pharmacological treatment is the first step in the management of all hypertensive patients, but it may be applied for anything from a few weeks to several years. During this time, cardiovascular damage may occur, leading to an increased risk of cardiovascular disease. Such

Multifactorial approach to the treatment of hypertension
• Lifestyle modification is recommended for all hypertensive individuals [2]
– for individuals with pre-hypertension it may prevent progression to hypertension
– changes to as many main modifiable causes (see Figure 2.2) as possible advocated for all individuals with hypertension, whether or not taking antihypertensive medication
• Antihypertensive medication(s)
– blood pressure control rates are poor in hypertensive patients who have been prescribed antihypertensive medication
– achieving target blood pressure depends on both efficacy of antihypertensive treatment and patient compliance [3]
– many patients who have been prescribed antihypertensive drug therapy do not adhere to their treatment regimen, or discontinue use within 1 year
– there are several potential causes of non-adherence to antihypertensive therapy (see Figure 3.11)

Figure 2.1 Multifactorial approach to the treatment of hypertension.

J. M. Neutel, *Combination Therapy in Hypertension*,
DOI: 10.1007/978-1-908517-28-9_2, © Springer Healthcare 2011

The main modifiable causes of hypertension
• Diet
– ideally, should be low in saturated fat, cholesterol, and total fat
– should be rich in potassium, magnesium, calcium, protein, and fiber
– increased consumption of fruit, vegetables, low-fat dairy products, whole grains, fish, poultry, and nuts is advocated
• High salt intake
– sodium reduction recommended for patients with high salt content in their diet
• Lack of exercise
– increasing aerobic exercise to 30–45 minutes per day is recommended
• Overweight/obesity
– assessing overall target weight and setting incremental weight loss targets may help patient focus on steady weight loss
• Excessive alcohol intake
– limitation of alcohol intake recommended; patients may require continuous support to ensure success
• Smoking
– smoking cessation advised; continuous monitoring and support may be required to ensure long-term success

Figure 2.2 The main modifiable causes of hypertension.

damage might have been prevented with earlier administration of pharmacological therapy.

Non-pharmacological treatment is considered by physicians to fail in the majority of patients because they are not compliant. Therefore, a better approach for the physician could be to prescribe antihypertensive medication from the time of initial diagnosis while also actively advocating a range of lifestyle modifications. Pharmacological treatment of hypertension represents a cost-effective way for preventing cardiovascular and renal complications [4].

Popularization of the stepped-care approach

The stepped-care approach to the management of hypertension comprises titration of initial monotherapy with antihypertensive drug, followed by addition of other antihypertensive medications with complementary modes of action, as necessary, to achieve blood pressure control (Figure 2.3). The concept of stepped care in the treatment of hypertension was devised in the 1960s when it became apparent that many hypertensive patients were not treated systematically to normotensive blood pressure levels [5]. The first Joint National Committee Report on Detection, Evaluation and Treatment of High

Stepped-care approach to the management of hypertension

1. Monotherapy is initiated with a low dose of antihypertensive drug

2. Dose of antihypertensive drug is increased in an attempt to achieve blood pressure control

3. Antihypertensive drug is substituted or new antihypertensive(s) added until blood pressure control is achieved

Figure 2.3 Stepped-care approach to the management of hypertension.

Blood Pressure published the stepped-care approach in 1977 [6], and this committee has advocated it for the management of hypertension ever since. The principle of the stepped-care approach is to treat people with a chronic illness with as few drugs as possible at the lowest doses possible. It has been described as a simple approach that enables individualization [5], and has been the preferred strategy for managing hypertension [7–9]. An algorithm for stepped-care treatment of hypertension is shown in Figure 2.4 [10].

Monotherapy is inadequate for blood pressure control in the majority of hypertensive patients [2,7]. Hypertension is a complex, multifactorial disease (see Chapter 1); therefore, the interruption of a single physiological pathway is often insufficient to normalize blood pressure in hypertensive patients. The percentage of hypertensive patients who achieve meaningful blood pressure control (responders) ranges from 30% to 60% with any class of drug given as monotherapy (Figure 2.5). The remaining patients will require a combination of at least two (and perhaps as many as four) antihypertensive drugs to achieve blood pressure control.

One of the factors that contribute to poor blood pressure control is the reluctance of physicians to titrate antihypertensive medication (see Figure 2.5). Physicians may accept slightly elevated blood pressures (i.e. inadequate blood pressure control) in treated hypertensive patients rather than titrating medication, changing drugs or adding another drug. This reluctance by physicians to change the treatment regimens may be explained by concerns about increased incidence of adverse events and adverse metabolic consequences with increased dose, higher cost, and patient resistance to polypharmacy and/or higher doses of medication. Also, physicians may be reluctant to add a second antihypertensive drug to the treatment regimen because there are few data available on the efficacy of the second drug in terms of blood pressure lowering, the prevention of hard outcomes, and the incidence of cardiovascular disease [11]. Choosing which second drug to add to initial therapy is, therefore, largely empirical and is not based on the best standards of evidence-based medicine [11]. As blood pressure control with monotherapy

Algorithm for stepped-care treatment of hypertension

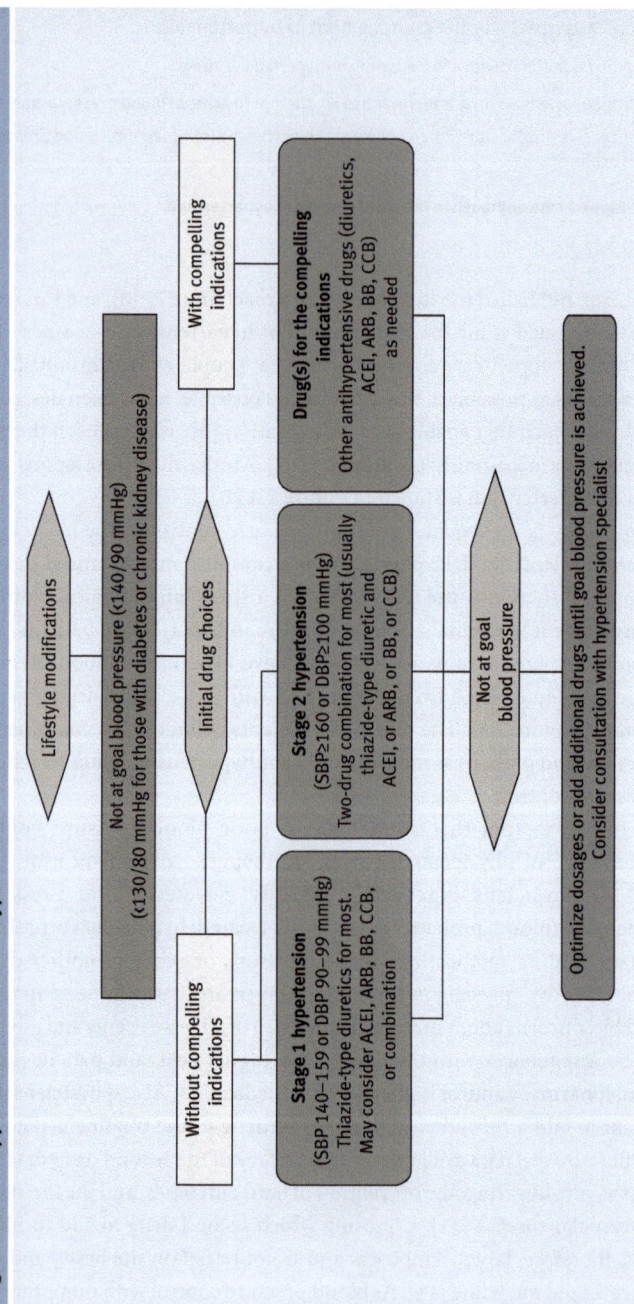

Figure 2.4 Algorithm for stepped-care treatment of hypertension. ACEI, angiotensin-converting enzyme inhibitor; ARB, angiotensin II receptor blocker; BB, β blocker; CCB, calcium channel blocker; DBP, diastolic blood pressure; SBP, systolic blood pressure. Reproduced with permission from Chobanian AV, Bakris GL, Black HR et al, The Seventh Report of the Joint National Committee on Prevention, Detection, Evaluation, and Treatment of High Blood Pressure: the JNC 7 report. JAMA 2003;289(19):2560–72.

Estimated efficacy of monotherapy in the treatment of hypertension	
Drug	Responders (%)
Thiazides	50–55
β Blockers	45–50
Angiotension-converting enzyme inhibitors	50–60
Calcium channel blockers	40–60
α Blockers (prazosin)	35–40
Central agonists	30–35

Figure 2.5 **Estimated efficacy of monotherapy in the treatment of hypertension.**
Reproduced with permission from Neutel JM. The use of combination drug therapy
in the treatment of hypertension. Prog Cardiovasc Nurs 2002; 17(2):81–8. Data
derived from Chobanian AV. Effects of beta blockers and other antihypertensive
drugs on cardiovascular risk. Am J Cardiol 1987; 59(13):48–52F.

is very difficult or impossible to achieve in the majority of patients, and as
physicians often will not titrate for inadequately controlled blood pressure,
the stepped-care approach may result in a significant number of hypertensive
patients being inadequately controlled. Indeed, current control rates for hypertension indicate that this approach is insufficiently effective in the management
of hypertension [12].

The rationale for the stepped-care approach in the treatment of hypertension
has been based mainly on the assumptions that monotherapy is more convenient
than combination therapy, is associated with fewer side effects, enables easier
identification of the drug causing an adverse event if one occurs, and is less
expensive. These assumptions are incorrect [7] (see Chapter 3).

Fixed-dose combination therapy

Although monotherapy is often the preferred choice for initiating treatment
of hypertension, this approach is only modestly effective in many patients
and target blood pressure goals are often not reached [13]. There is increasing
awareness that the elusive goal of a 'normal' blood pressure is achieved only
if multiple drug therapy is used [14]. Most hypertensive patients require the
co-administration of two or more drugs from different therapeutic classes to
achieve a blood pressure of less than 140/90 mmHg [15].

There are two options for multiple drug therapy in the treatment of hypertension: one option, the stepped-care approach, is to add drugs sequentially until
an effective multiple drug regimen is achieved (see above); the other option is
fixed-dose combination therapy. Fixed-dose combination drugs combine two
agents at each of the highest recommended doses into one tablet for convenience.

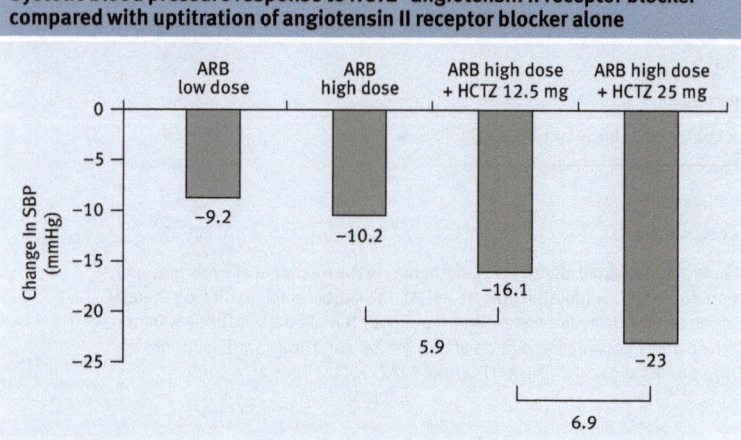

Figure 2.6 Systolic blood pressure response to HCTZ–angiotensin II receptor blocker compared with uptitration of angiotensin II receptor blocker alone. ARB, angiotensin II receptor blocker; HCTZ, hydrochlorothiazide; SBP, systolic blood pressure. Reproduced with permission from Neutel JM. The role of combination therapy in the management of hypertension. Nephrol Dial Transplant 2006; 21(6):1469–74.

These are clearly distinguishable from low-dose combination drugs, which use low doses of each component drug to provide additive hypotensive effects with relatively few side effects. High-dose fixed combinations have become more popular with the introduction of well-tolerated drugs that have complimentary side effect profiles such as high dose angiotensin II receptor blocker (ARB) with hydrochlorothiazide (HCTZ) – HCTZ is potassium losing, ARBs are potassium sparing, and the net result is no change in potassium.

The concept of fixed-dose combination therapy was developed in the 1950s [14] and this treatment approach has been used since the 1960s [16]. The rationale behind fixed-dose combination therapy has remained constant since this approach was developed [14,17–21]:

- Two drugs, each typically working at a separate site, block different effector pathways; therefore, blood pressure-lowering effect may be enhanced when two drug classes are co-administered.
- One of the drugs may counteract counter-regulatory mechanisms that are triggered by the other drug, thereby potentially improving efficacy.
- Combination therapy is often associated with fewer adverse effects than high-dose monotherapy, which may lead to improved patient compliance.

- One component of a fixed-dose combination therapy may effectively neutralize some of the adverse effects of the other component.
- Simplicity of administration of fixed-dose combination therapy may improve compliance; thereby, preventing treatment failures that might result from missed doses.

Fixed-dose combination antihypertensive therapy has been available for almost a half-century. During that time, considerable progress has been made in the development of physiologically appropriate combinations [22]. Fixed-dose combination therapy has a proven record of reducing blood pressure. Many physicians have used fixed-dose combination therapy even when academic approval and enthusiasm for this therapeutic approach were lacking [14]. Fixed-dose combinations are becoming increasingly popular as physicians realize that bringing patients to blood pressure goal quickly is likely to improve clinical outcomes.

The inadequate control of systolic blood pressure is well known to be the major factor contributing to poor rates of blood pressure control. Systolic hypertension is volume dependent and, therefore, very responsive to diuretics. However, high doses of diuretics are associated with adverse events and metabolic adverse effects; therefore, the maximal dose of the diuretic, HCTZ, that should be administered to a hypertensive patient is generally agreed to be 12.5 mg. Nevertheless, many new combination drugs contain HCTZ at a 25 mg dose. The reasons for this are exemplified in Figure 2.6. This shows that uptitration of an ARB from a low dose to a high dose causes only a slight further reduction in systolic blood pressure, i.e. this drug has a flat dose–response curve. In contrast, the addition of HCTZ 12.5 mg to the high-dose ARB causes a very impressive further reduction in systolic blood pressure [23]. The addition of a further 12.5 mg HCTZ (total 25 mg HCTZ) may be expected to result in a flat dose–response curve; however, the additional 12.5 mg HCTZ causes a further decrease that is similar to that with the initial 12.5 mg [24]. This further decrease in systolic blood pressure is not unexpected, given that systolic hypertension is volume dependent and, therefore, very responsive to diuretics. The adverse event profile with high-dose fixed ARB and HCTZ combination therapy is similar to that with high-dose HCTZ monotherapy [25]. The complementary nature of these agents enables greater reductions in systolic blood pressure without substantially impacting the adverse event profile.

Simplification of the antihypertensive drug regimen is critical for the effective management of hypertension. Addition of antihypertensive drugs to a treatment regimen has been shown to significantly decrease compliance with treatment, even if the drugs are given once daily [25]. However, use of a fixed-dose combination therapy simplifies the dosing regimen and is associated with improved compliance rates compared with monotherapy. Blood pressure control is achieved more rapidly with combination therapy compared with monotherapy (even at high doses), and this improves patient compliance and decreases the incidence of cardiovascular disease.

Low-dose combination therapy

The aim of low-dose combination therapy is to achieve blood pressure control with small doses of each agent, thereby eliciting fewer dose-dependent adverse effects than would be seen with higher doses of either agent as monotherapy. The concept of low-dose combination therapy arose mainly from experience with diuretics, which are useful in combination with other classes of antihypertensive drugs because they reduce the fluid retention often associated with vasodilators. Thiazide diuretics were initially prescribed, and were very effective, in high doses (at least 100 mg), but they were associated with many metabolic side effects and other adverse events. Lower doses of diuretics were shown still to provide blood pressure control, but with an improved adverse metabolic effect profile and adverse event profile. Most adverse effects with diuretics were, therefore, shown to be dose dependent. Diuretics are increasingly being prescribed in low-dose combination therapies to provide blood pressure control with minimal side effects.

As physicians recognize that most patients with hypertension require combination therapy to achieve blood pressure goals, fixed-dose preparations are becoming increasingly popular in clinical practice [26,27]. The inclusion of fixed-dose preparations, preferably fixed low-dose combinations, as a first-line option for the treatment of hypertension in hypertension guidelines in the USA and Europe has also widened their acceptance and increased their popularity [20]. Greater use of combination therapy has been associated with an increase in control rates.

References

1. Trotman BW. Hypertension: a multietiological disease requires a multifactorial approach. J Assoc Acad Minor Phys 1995; 6(4):124.

2. Whitworth JA; World Health Organization, International Society of Hypertension Writing Group. 2003 World Health Organization (WHO)/International Society of Hypertension (ISH) statement on management of hypertension. J Hypertens 2003; 21(11):1983–92.

3. Unger T, McInnes GT, Neutel JM, Böhm M. The role of olmesartan medoxomil in the management of hypertension. Drugs 2004; 64(24):2731–9.

4. Struijker-Boudier AJ, Ambrosioni E, Holzgreve H, et al. The need for combination antihypertensive therapy to reach target blood pressures: what has been learned from clinical practice and morbidity-mortality trials? Int J Clin Pract 2007; 61(9):1592–602.

5. Moser M. Is the stepped-care approach to the management of hypertension still appropriate? Chest 1985; 88(4):629.

6. Report of the Joint National Committee on Detection, Evaluation and Treatment of High Blood Pressure. A cooperative study. JAMA 1977; 237:255–61.

7. Neutel JM. The use of combination drug therapy in the treatment of hypertension. Prog Cardiovasc Nurs 2002; 17(2):81–8.

8. Fahey T, Schroeder K, Ebrahim S. Educational and organisational interventions used to improve the management of hypertension in primary care: a systematic review. Br J Gen Pract 2005; 55(520):875–82.

9. Fahey T, Schroeder K, Ebrahim S. Interventions used to improve control of blood pressure in patients with hypertension. Cochrane Database Syst Rev 2006; (4):CD005182.

10. The Seventh Report of the Joint National Committee on Prevention, Detection, Evaluation, and Treatment of High Blood Pressure. US Department of Health and Human Services. NIH Publication No. 04-5230. Bethesda, MD: National Institutes of Health, August 2004.

11. Fuchs FD, Guerrero P, Gus M. What is next when the first blood pressure-lowering drug is not sufficient? Expert Rev Cardiovasc Ther 2007; 5(3):435–9.

12. Neutel JM. The role of combination therapy in the management of hypertension. Nephrol Dial Transplant 2006; 21(6):1469–74.

13. Sica DA. Rationale for fixed-dose combinations in the treatment of hypertension: the cycle repeats. Drugs 2002; 62:443–62.

14. Flack JM. Epidemiology and unmet needs in hypertension. J Manag Care Pharm 2007; 13(8 Suppl B):2–8.

15. Waeber B, Brunner HR. Rationale for the use of very-low-dose combinations as first-line treatment of hypertension. J Hypertens Suppl 2001; 19:S3–8.

16. Weir MR, Bakris GL. Combination therapy with renin–angiotensin-aldosterone receptor blockers for hypertension: how far have we come? J Clin Hypertens (Greenwich) 2008; 10:146–52.

17. Waeber B. Combination therapy with ACE inhibitors/angiotensin II receptor antagonists and diuretics in hypertension. Expert Rev Cardiovasc Ther 2003; 1:43–50.

18. Giles TD. Rationale for combination therapy as initial treatment for hypertension. J Clin Hypertens (Greenwich) 2003; 5(4 Suppl 3):4–11.

19. Weir MR. When antihypertensive monotherapy fails: fixed-dose combination therapy. South Med J 2000; 93(6):548–56.

20. Epstein M, Bakris G. Newer approaches to antihypertensive therapy. Use of fixed-dose combination therapy. Arch Intern Med 1996; 156:1969–78.

21. Ménard J. Critical assessment of combination therapy development. Blood Press Suppl 1993; 1:5–9.

22. Sica DA. Fixed-dose combination antihypertensive drugs. Do they have a role in rational therapy? Drugs 1994; 48:16–24.

23. Neutel JM, Saunders E, Bakris GL, et al., INCLUSIVE Investigators. The efficacy and safety of low- and high-dose fixed combinations of irbesartan/hydrochlorothiazide in patients with uncontrolled systolic blood pressure on monotherapy: the INCLUSIVE trial. J Clin Hypertens 2005; 7(10):578–86.

24. Kochar M, Guthrie R, Triscari J, Kassler-Taub K, Reeves RA. Matrix study of irbesartan with hydrochlorothiazide in mild-to-moderate hypertension. Am J Hypertens 1999; 12:797–805.

25. Mancia G, Omboni S, Grassi G. Combination treatment in hypertension: the VeraTran study. Am J Hypertens 1997; 10:153S–158S.

26. Coca A, Calvo C, Sobrino J, et al. Once-daily fixed-combination irbesartan 300 mg/ hydrochlorothiazide 25 mg and circadian blood pressure profile in patients with essential hypertension. Clin Ther 2003; 25:2849 –64.

27. Neutel JM, Franklin SS, Oparil S, Bhaumik A, Ptaszynska A, Lapuerta P. Efficacy and safety of irbesartan/HCTZ combination therapy as initial treatment for rapid control of severe hypertension. J Clin Hypertens 2006; 8:850–7; quiz 858–9.

Chapter 3

Advantages of combination therapy compared with monotherapy

Properties of the ideal antihypertensive agent are given in Figure 3.1. These properties are difficult to achieve with monotherapy; therefore, low doses of complementary drugs have been combined in an attempt to create a treatment for hypertension that is closer to the ideal. Administration of two complementary antihypertensive drugs in combination is always associated with greater efficacy than uptitration of an individual antihypertensive agent and provides an improved adverse event profile compared with monotherapy.

This chapter details the advantages of combination therapy compared with monotherapy.

Efficacy

Administration of a combination of two complementary antihypertensive drugs in low doses is well known to cause an additive reduction in both systolic and diastolic blood pressure. For example, the mean decrease in diastolic blood pressure with low-dose amlodipine–benazepril combination

Properties of the ideal antihypertensive agent
• Effective in reduction of blood pressure
• Effective over 24 hours with once-a-day dosing
• High response rate; works well in all subgroups of hypertensive patients
• No/reduced side effects
• No/reduced negative metabolic side effects
• End-organ protection beyond blood pressure control
• Affordable (reduces the cost of treating the patient)

Figure 3.1 Properties of the ideal antihypertensive agent.

J. M. Neutel, *Combination Therapy in Hypertension*,
DOI: 10.1007/978-1-908517-28-9_3, © Springer Healthcare 2011

Mean decreases in diastolic blood pressure with low-dose amlodipine, benazepril, and amlodipine–benazepril combination therapy

Treatment	Mean decrease in diastolic blood pressure (mmHg)*	Response rate (% patients)
Placebo	–	15.8
Amlodipine 5 mg	8.6	67.5
Benazepril 20 mg	7.0	53.3
Amlodipine 5 mg–benazepril 20 mg	13.9	87.0
*Placebo subtracted		

Figure 3.2 **Mean decreases in diastolic blood pressure with low-dose amlodipine, benazepril, and amlodipine–benazepril combination therapy.** Reproduced with permission from Neutel JM. The use of combination drug therapy in the treatment of hypertension. Prog Cardiovasc Nurs 2002; 17(2):81–8. Data from Clin Ther 1996; 1B:6–12.

therapy (13.9 mmHg) is greater than that with either amlodipine alone (8.6 mmHg) or benazepril alone (7.0 mmHg) (Figure 3.2).

As well as being greater than that of each of the components alone, the reduction in blood pressure with two low-dose complementary antihypertensive drugs is usually greater than with significantly higher doses of each of the components alone. Figure 3.3 shows that a low dose of hydrochlorothiazide (HCTZ; 6.25 mg)

Decreases in diastolic blood pressure with hydrochlorothiazide, bisoprolol and hydrochlorothiazide–bisoprolol combination therapy

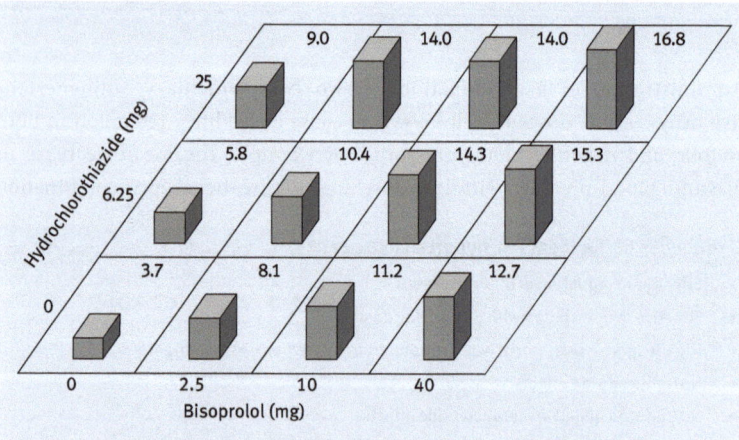

Figure 3.3 **Decreases in diastolic blood pressure with hydrochlorothiazide, bisoprolol and hydrochlorothiazide–bisoprolol combination therapy.** Reproduced with permission from Neutel JM. The role of combination therapy in the management of hypertension. Nephrol Dial Transplant 2006; 21(6):1469–74.

used in combination with a low dose of bisoprolol (10 mg) is more efficacious in reducing diastolic blood pressure from baseline than high-dose HCTZ mono-therapy (25 mg) or high-dose bisoprolol monotherapy (40 mg) [1,2]. Similarly, Figure 3.4 shows that addition of a low dose of HCTZ (12.5 mg) to a low dose of angiotensin II receptor blocker (ARB) causes a greater decrease in systolic blood pressure than uptitrating the dose of ARB monotherapy [1,3,4].

These results indicate that the efficacy achieved with complementary anti-hypertensive drugs in combination may be as much as threefold greater than that achieved with uptitration of monotherapy. As hypertension is a multisys-tem disease (see Chapter 1), it follows that the interruption of more than one system with a combination of complementary drugs is more likely to reduce blood pressure than aggressive blockade of only one system. Low-dose com-bination therapy provides novel coverage of two or more metabolic pathways that contribute to hypertension.

The response rate to any single class of drug given as monotherapy ranges from 30% to 60% (see Figure 2.5); however, this rate increases to 75–95% using a combination of two complementary antihypertensive drugs. In contrast to monotherapy, low-dose combination therapy enables blood pressure control to

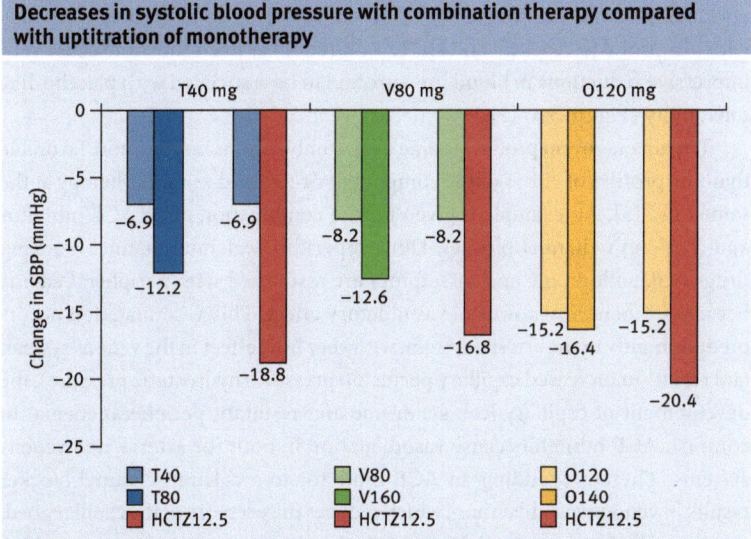

Figure 3.4 Decreases in systolic blood pressure with combination therapy compared with uptitration of monotherapy. HCTZ, hydrochlorothiazide; O, olmesartan; SBP, systolic blood pressure; T, telmisartan; V, valsartan. Reproduced with permission from Neutel JM. The role of combination therapy in the management of hypertension. Nephrol Dial Transplant 2006; 21(6):1469–74.

be achieved in all subgroups of hypertensive patients (hence there is a higher response rate with combination therapy) (see Chapter 4).

Safety

The adverse effect profile with monotherapy for the treatment of hypertension is generally assumed to be better than that with combination therapy; however, this is not the case. Monotherapy is frequently associated with more side effects than low-dose combination therapy. Only around half of patients who receive monotherapy will achieve blood pressure control. Of these responding patients, around 60–70% will require the highest recommended dose of monotherapy to achieve blood pressure control.

Most of the adverse events associated with antihypertensive treatment are dose dependent (except for angiotensin-converting enzyme [ACE] inhibitor-induced cough), which means that patients who are receiving high doses of monotherapy are more likely to experience drug-related side effects than patients treated and controlled on low-dose combination therapy. The lower risk of adverse effects with low-dose combination therapy supports the increased interest in a more combined approach to the treatment of hypertension. For example, although β blockers and diuretics have many dose-dependent side effects that can be limiting at high doses, a low-dose combination of therapy with bisoprolol (β blocker) and HCTZ (diuretic) has been shown to cause very impressive reductions in blood pressure and to be associated with placebo-like tolerability (Figure 3.5) [2].

The adverse event profile of some drug combinations may be more favorable than the profiles of either of the component drugs used as monotherapy at the same dose [5]. An example is given for the combination of an ACE inhibitor and a calcium channel blocker. Dihydropyridine calcium channel blocking drugs (e.g. amlodipine and nifedipine) are associated with peripheral edema because of their very powerful vasodilatory effect. This vasodilatation occurs predominantly in the arterial system, with very little effect in the venous system, and results in increased capillary perfusion pressure (hydrostatic pressure), the development of capillary leak syndrome and resultant peripheral edema. In contrast, ACE inhibitors cause vasodilatation in both the arterial and venous systems. Therefore, adding an ACE inhibitor to a calcium channel blocker results in venous vasodilatation, which reduces the pressure in the capillary bed, thereby reducing the potential for peripheral edema. A simple diagram to show the pathogenesis of vasodilatory edema is given in Figure 3.6. The combination therapy results in less edema than similar doses of the calcium channel blocker given as monotherapy, despite greater reduction in blood pressure [5].

Placebo-like adverse event profile with low-dose combination therapy		
	Placebo (n=144)	Bisoprolol 2.5 mg– HCTZ 10 mg (n=221)
BP reduction (mmHg)	2.9/3.9	15.8/12.6
Adverse event (%)		
Bradycardia	0.7	0.9
Peripheral ischemia	0.9	0.4
Bronchospasm	0.0	0.0
Cough	0.7	3.0
Dizziness	1.8	3.2
Headache	2.7	0.4
Insomnia	2.0	1.2
Somnolence	0.7	0.9
Loss of libido	1.2	0.4
Impotence	0.7	1.1

Figure 3.5 Placebo-like adverse event profile with low-dose combination therapy.
BP, blood pressure; HCTZ, hydrochlorothiazide. Reproduced with permission from
Neutel JM. The role of combination therapy in the management of hypertension.
Nephrol Dial Transplant 2006; 21(6):1469–74.

According to surveys of physicians, the efficacy and safety of antihypertensive drugs are the most important qualities to consider when selecting initial drugs for treatment of hypertension [1]. Increasing the dose of an antihypertensive drug given as monotherapy is associated with increased efficacy, but also with increased dose-dependent side effects, i.e. efficacy and safety are opposed. In contrast, increasing the dose of combination therapy is associated with greater efficacy, but not necessarily at the expense of safety, i.e. efficacy and safety are aligned towards the ideal antihypertensive (Figure 3.7).

It has been suggested that a disadvantage of combination therapy, compared with monotherapy, is that it in the presence of an adverse event it is more difficult to identify the drug that is causing the problem. However, it is usually obvious which antihypertensive agent is responsible for an adverse event, even when the drug is used as part of a combination. For example, if a patient who is taking ACE inhibitor monotherapy develops a chronic dry cough, the cough will be determined to be in response to ACE inhibition. If a patient who is taking a combination of an ACE inhibitor and a calcium channel blocker develops a chronic dry cough, it is clear that this adverse effect is because of the ACE inhibitor. If a side effect develops in a patient who was started on low-dose combination therapy, the combination agent could be as easily discontinued as a monotherapeutic agent.

Pathogenesis of vasodilatory edema

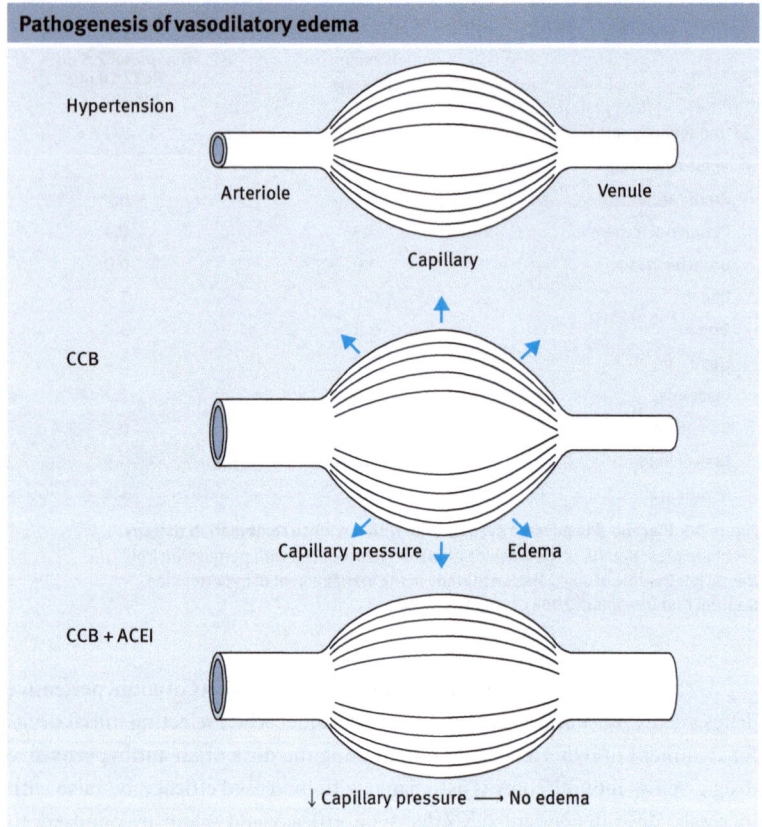

Figure 3.6 Pathogenesis of vasodilatory edema. ACEI, angiotensin-converting enzyme inhibitor; CCB, calcium channel blocker.

Cost

The overall cost of treating hypertension is often assumed to equate simply to the cost of the antihypertensive drug. This assumption is incorrect: several factors contribute to the overall cost of treating hypertension (Figure 3.8). The overall cost of treating hypertension, therefore, should be calculated as the cost of treating the patient, not the cost of individual drugs [5]. For example, it may not always be cost-effective to prescribe the cheapest available antihypertensive therapies. Administration of a slightly more expensive antihypertensive agent that is well tolerated by patients, rather than a cheaper less well-tolerated drug, may decrease the overall cost of treating hypertension by reducing office visits and decreasing the incidence of drug-related adverse events. That said, in high-risk patients who

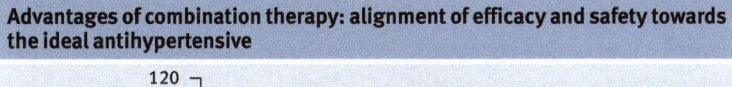

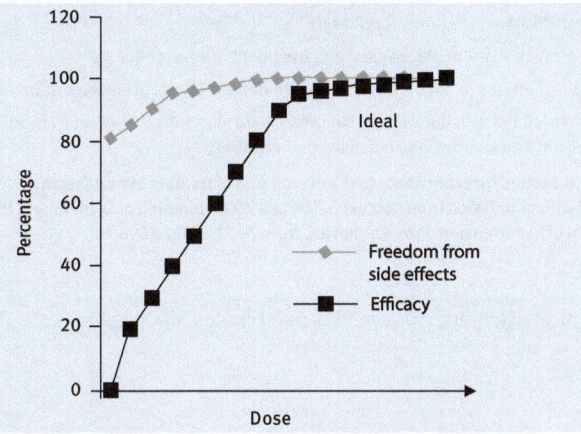

Figure 3.7 Advantages of combination therapy: alignment of efficacy and safety towards the ideal antihypertensive. Reproduced with permission from Neutel JM. The role of combination therapy in the management of hypertension. Nephrol Dial Transplant 2006; 21(6):1469–74.

attain large benefits from treatment, expensive drugs may be cost-effective, but in low-risk patients, treatment may not be cost-effective unless the drugs are cheap [6]. Successful treatment of hypertension, i.e. achieving adequate blood pressure control with minimal side effects, is associated with significant costs; however, uncontrolled hypertension is also costly in terms of increased office visits (Figure 3.9).

'Two-drug monotherapy,' a regimen comprising two monotherapeutic agents prescribed at the same time, is often the most expensive regimen for treating hypertension because many office visits are required for drug titration, and using two agents is obviously associated with two dispensing fees, two co-payments, and the cost of two drugs. Each of the high-dose monotherapies that it consists of sometimes requires two tablets or capsules of a particular drug per dose, which doubles the cost of medication. In contrast, low-dose combination therapy comprises use of a combination agent that is slightly more expensive than each of the component drugs alone, but cheaper than if each drug was used separately in a combination treatment regimen. Also, using one combination agent is associated with only one dispensing fee and one co-payment. Thus, low-dose combination therapy is cheaper than two-drug monotherapy (Figure 3.10) [8], and is often cheaper than high-dose monotherapy with either component drug.

Factors that contribute to the overall cost of treating hypertension

- Cost of antihypertensive medication
- Cost of office visits required for titration
- Cost of office visits for assessment and treatment of adverse events
- Cost of laboratory tests to assess adverse metabolic effects of antihypertensive medication
- Cost associated with the increased mortality and morbidity that result from poor patient compliance and inadequate blood pressure control

Figure 3.8 Factors that contribute to the overall cost of treating hypertension.
Adapted with permission from Neutel JM. The use of combination drug therapy in the treatment of hypertension. Prog Cardiovasc Nurs 2002; 17(2):81–8.

Uncontrolled hypertension results in increased office visits

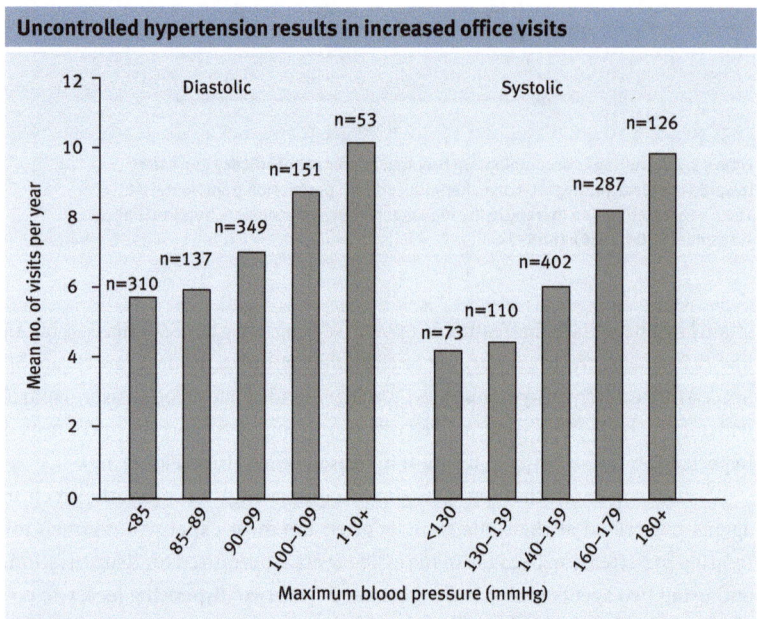

Figure 3.9 Uncontrolled hypertension results in increased office visits. Data from [7].

Compliance

Poor compliance is the most important reason for inadequate blood pressure control in hypertensive patients (see Figure 1.4) and may be the result of several factors (Figure 3.11). As shown in Figure 3.11, the two most important factors that influence patient compliance with antihypertensive treatment are real and perceived drug-related adverse events (see earlier) and convenience of the antihypertensive drug dosing schedule (Figure 3.12). The many low-dose

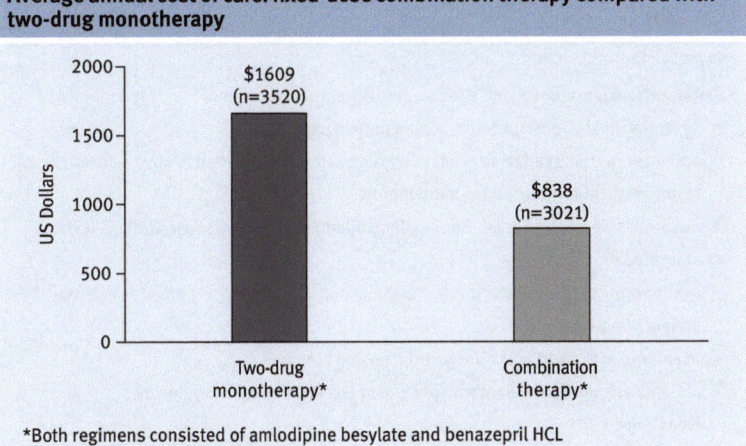

Average annual cost of care: fixed-dose combination therapy compared with two-drug monotherapy

*Both regimens consisted of amlodipine besylate and benazepril HCL

Figure 3.10 Average annual cost of care: fixed-dose combination therapy compared with two-drug monotherapy. Data from [8].

combination antihypertensive therapies that are available are in single tablet or capsule form, and are taken once daily, which makes combination therapy as convenient to the patient as monotherapy [5,9]. Furthermore, blood pressure has a circadian pattern with a rapid morning surge that is associated with an increased risk of myocardial infarction, unstable angina, stroke, and sudden cardiac death. Therefore, greater cardiovascular benefits may be attainable if antihypertensive drugs administered once daily maintain blood pressure control throughout the 24-hour dosing period, including the high-risk early morning hours.

An important advantage of low-dose combination therapy is that antihypertensive agents can be incorporated into the combination agent at doses much lower than could be obtained with commercially available monotherapeutic agents. To achieve very low doses with monotherapeutic agents would require accurate drug splitting: most patients, particularly the elderly, would not be able to manage this, and compliance would be affected.

Patients with hypertension are generally resistant to polypharmacy [9]. The prescription of multiple drugs makes them feel as if they have a more severe illness than they realized, and the complicated multiple-drug-dosing regimen may be confusing for them and affect their compliance with treatment. The use of combination therapy decreases polypharmacy, which results in improved compliance.

Factors that may influence patient compliance with antihypertensive treatment

Two most important factors

- Antihypertensive drug-related adverse events (real and perceived)
  - by far the most important cause of poor patient compliance
  - patients may report adverse event to physician, but may respond to adverse event by not taking medication or by taking it irregularly
  - nearly all side effects are dose dependent: administering lower doses often alleviates side effects
  - the importance of side effects in the management of hypertensive patients is often underestimated
- Convenience of the antihypertensive drug dosing schedule
  - patients are more compliant with once-daily than with twice-daily dosing (see Figure 3.12)
  - drug-splitting is likely to have a negative impact on compliance
  - patients are generally resistant to polypharmacy
  - the greater the number of changes made to treatment in an attempt to achieve blood pressure control, the poorer the compliance

Other factors

- Patient's inadequate knowledge/incomplete understanding of disease/treatment
- Little input/interest from the patient with regard to treatment program
- Denial of illness
- Lack of symptoms
- Impact on quality of life
- Failure of physicians to be aggressive enough in achieving adequate blood pressure control
- Cultural or socioeconomic factors
- Cost of drugs and other costs associated with management of hypertension (see Figure 3.8)

Figure 3.11 Factors that may influence patient compliance with antihypertensive treatment. BP, blood pressure; HCTZ, hydrochlorothiazide.

Effectiveness of antihypertensive treatment depends not only on the drugs avoiding or minimizing symptomatic side effects but also on them having a positive effect on quality of life [10]. Controlling blood pressure appears to be an important element in improving subjective health perceptions of hypertensive patients [10]. Any real or perceived negative effects of antihypertensive therapy on sexual function and other aspects of quality of life may impact on compliance with treatment. In this respect, it is worth noting that combination therapy (bisoprolol–HCTZ) has been reported to be no more likely to be associated with

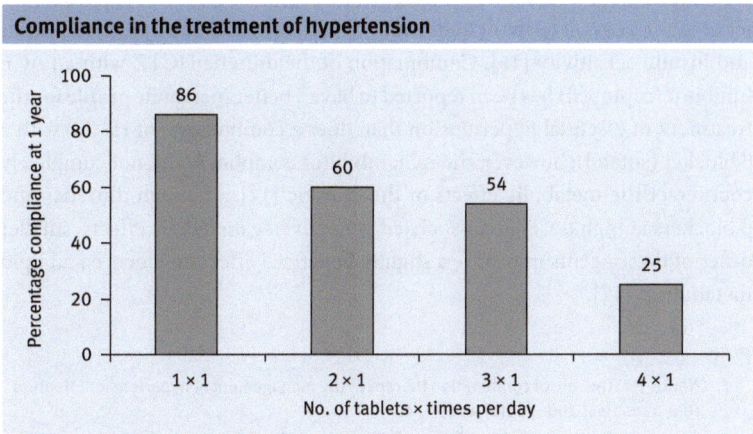

Compliance in the treatment of hypertension

Figure 3.12 Compliance in the treatment of hypertension.

sexual dysfunction than placebo or monotherapy (HCTZ, bisoprolol, enalapril, or amlodipine) in hypertensive patients [11].

Improving patient compliance is a major goal in the management of hypertension [12]. To achieve this goal, several issues need to be addressed, including safety, convenience, patient preference [13], and the level of patient involvement in their treatment. Convincing patients of the efficacy of antihypertensive therapy as early as possible during treatment is also likely to improve patient compliance.

Metabolic effects

Diuretics and β blockers, when administered at high doses, negatively impact on lipid metabolism and insulin sensitivity, whereas ACE inhibitors and calcium antagonists tend to have little effect on these metabolic risk factors [14]. Metabolic side effects of antihypertensive drugs may increase the risk of coronary artery disease despite an adequate reduction in blood pressure [15]. The metabolic side effects associated with antihypertensive therapy tend to be dose dependent; for example, the hypokalemia and hyperglycemia associated with thiazide diuretics, and the reduction in high-density lipoprotein-cholesterol with some β blockers, are dose dependent [5]. The use of combination therapies with low doses of antihypertensive agents minimizes the risk of metabolic adverse effects while significantly reducing blood pressure. For example, a study in non-obese, normolipidemic, glucose-tolerant, hypertensive patients showed that normalization of blood pressure by means of a daily combination therapy (verapamil 180 mg–trandolapril 2 mg or atenolol 50 mg–nifedipine 20 mg) is feasible at no cost in terms of undesired effects on glucose and lipid metabolism and insulin sensitivity [16]. Combination of the diuretic HCTZ with an ACE inhibitor (captopril) has been reported to have a better metabolic profile for the treatment of essential hypertension than does a combination of HCTZ with a β blocker (sotalol); however, the ACE inhibitor component did not completely counteract the metabolic effects of the diuretic [14]. Although diuretics and β blockers at high doses are associated with adverse metabolic effects, smaller doses of these agents may have a slightly beneficial effect on glucose and lipid metabolism [17].

References

1. Neutel JM. The role of combination therapy in the management of hypertension. Nephrol Dial Transplant 2006; 21(6):1469–74.

2. Frishman WH, Bryzinski BS, Coulson LR, et al. A multifactorial trial design to assess combination therapy in hypertension. Treatment with bisoprolol and hydrochlorothiazide. Arch Intern Med 1994; 154:1461–8.

3. Kochar M, Guthrie R, Triscari J, Kassler-Taub K, Reeves RA. Matrix study of irbesartan with hydrochlorothiazide in mild-to-moderate hypertension. Am J Hypertens 1999; 12:797–805.

4. Chrysant SG, Weber MA, Wang AC, Hinman DJ. Evaluation of antihypertensive therapy with the combination of olmesartan medoxomil and hydrochlorothiazide. Am J Hypertens 2004; 17:252–9.

5. Neutel JM. The use of combination drug therapy in the treatment of hypertension. Prog Cardiovasc Nurs 2002; 17(2):81–8.

6. Whitworth JA; World Health Organization, International Society of Hypertension Writing Group. 2003 World Health Organization (WHO)/International Society of Hypertension (ISH) statement on management of hypertension. J Hypertens 2003; 21(11):1983–92.

7. Paramore LC, Halpern MT, Lapuerta P, et al. Impact of poorly controlled hypertension on healthcare resource utilization and cost. Am J Manag Care 2001; 7:389–98.

8. Taylor AA, Shoheiber O. Adherence to antihypertensive therapy with fixed-dose amlodipine besylate/benazepril HCl versus comparable component-based therapy. Congest Heart Fail 2003; 9:324–32.

9. Neutel JM Combination therapy and the treatment of hypertension. Cardiology Special Edition 2003; 9(1 of 2):11–15.

10. Weber MA, Bakris GL, Neutel JM, Davidai G, Giles TD. Quality of life measured in a practice-based hypertension trial of an angiotensin receptor blocker. J Clin Hypertens 2003; 5(5):322–9.

11. Prisant LM, Weir MR, Frishman WH, Neutel JM, Davidov ME, Lewin AJ. Self reported sexual dysfunction in men and women treated with bisoprolol, hydrochlorothiazide, enalapril, amlodipine, placebo, or bisoprolol/hydrochlorothiazide. J Clin Hypertens 1999; 1(1):22–6.

12. Neutel JM, Smith DH. Improving patient compliance: a major goal in the management of hypertension. J Clin Hypertens 2003; 5(2):127–32.

13. Montgomery AA, Harding J, Fahey T. Shared decision making in hypertension: the impact of patient preferences on treatment choice. Fam Pract 2001; 18(3):309–13.

14. Neutel JM. Metabolic manifestations of low-dose diuretics. Am J Med 1996; 101(3A): 71S–82S.

15. Middeke M, Richter WO, Schwandt P, Holzgreve H. The effects of antihypertensive combination therapy on lipid and glucose metabolism: hydrochlorothiazide plus sotalol vs. hydrochlorothiazide plus captopril. Int J Clin Pharmacol Ther 1997; 35(6):231–4.

16. Quiñones-Galvan A, Pucciarelli A, Ciociaro D, Masoni A, Franzoni F, Natali A, Ferrannini E. Metabolic effects of combined antihypertensive treatment in patients with essential hypertension. J Cardiovasc Pharmacol 2002; 40(6):916–21.

17. Neutel JM, Rolf CN, Valentine SN, Li J, Lucus C, Marmorstein BL. Low-dose combination therapy as first line treatment of mild-to-moderate hypertension: the efficacy and safety of bisoprolol/HCTZ versus amlodipine, enalapril, and placebo. Cardiovasc Rev Rep 1996; 71:33–45.

Chapter 4

Use of combination therapy in special populations

Many different physiological factors contribute to the development of hypertension. The relative contribution of these factors varies between different population subgroups. As a result, the responsiveness of the subgroups to antihypertensive medications also varies. However, the results of clinical studies indicate that administration of low-dose combination therapy enables adequate blood pressure control to be achieved in all subgroups of hypertensive patients, including the elderly, African–Americans, Caucasians, and patients with diabetes or metabolic syndrome. Such an effect is not seen with monotherapy. Proven efficacy with low-dose combination therapy across a broad range of patient groups simplifies the treatment of hypertension: selection of combination therapy should enable physicians to achieve blood pressure control in most of their patients. Furthermore, achieving blood pressure control early in the course of treating hypertension is likely to motivate patients to remain compliant with their antihypertensive medication.

The elderly

Hypertension is a major risk factor for stroke and coronary events in elderly individuals. Treatment of hypertension in the elderly is associated with decreased rates of total mortality, cardiovascular mortality, and stroke; however, control of blood pressure in the elderly is poor [1]. Management of hypertension in elderly patients is complicated by several age-related factors, including physiological changes, co-morbid conditions, functional or cognitive impairments, and polypharmacy issues [2]:

- elderly patients with hypertension are more likely than younger patients with this condition to have developed organ damage related to hypertension or to have heart failure;

J. M. Neutel, *Combination Therapy in Hypertension*,
DOI: 10.1007/978-1-908517-28-9_4, © Springer Healthcare 2011

- high blood pressure raises the risks of vascular dementia and cognitive dysfunction in older adults [3];
- the elderly are often receiving multiple medications, which increases the risk for adverse drug interactions; and
- the elderly may be more likely to struggle to maintain compliance with complicated and/or additional drug regimens.

Furthermore, it has been suggested that physicians are generally less aggressive in controlling blood pressure in elderly than in younger patients [4].

Combination therapy is indicated for the majority of elderly patients with hypertension. For example, combination therapy with a calcium channel blocker and an angiotensin-converting enzyme (ACE) inhibitor (two classes of metabolically neutral agents) may effectively preserve cognitive function, as well as reducing blood pressure, with good tolerability [1]. The low-dose combination of the ACE inhibitor perindopril (2 mg) and the diuretic indapamide (0.625 mg) has been shown to result in sustained blood pressure control when used as first-line treatment of elderly hypertensive patients (aged 65–85 years) over 1 year, and to be well tolerated [5]. The good tolerability and simplified regimen associated with low-dose combination therapy may greatly improve compliance and control rates in elderly patients with hypertension.

African–Americans

Prevalence data for different racial or ethnic groups in the USA indicate that a disproportionate number of African–Americans have hypertension compared with non-Hispanic whites and Mexican–Americans [6,7]. African–Americans develop hypertension at an earlier age than Caucasians, their average blood pressures are much higher and they experience more severe disease, possibly as a result of the higher prevalence of concomitant cardiovascular risk factors in this population [7,8]. The earlier onset and greater severity of hypertension in African–Americans contribute to a greater burden of hypertensive target organ damage in this population (for example, they are at increased risk for left ventricular hypertrophy, heart failure, and end-stage renal disease compared with white individuals with hypertension [7,9]) and may be factors in the shorter life expectancy of this population compared with white Americans [6].

Cardiovascular mortality in African–Americans with hypertension is three- to five-times higher than in Caucasians with hypertension, and African–American hypertensives tend to progress more frequently to end-stage renal disease and stroke [10]. The results of a study of the level of medical care provided to African–American and Caucasian patients with hypertension do not explain disparities in hypertension-related outcomes between these patient populations [11]. The increased prevalence of hypertension and excessive target organ damage among African–Americans is because of a combination of genetic and, most likely, environmental factors. There is a clear need for improved management of hypertension in African–Americans via therapeutic lifestyle interventions and pharmacotherapy [6].

Monotherapy with diuretics or calcium channel blockers is relatively more effective at lowering blood pressure in African–Americans than are ACE inhibitors, angiotensin II receptor blockers (ARBs), and β blockers. Indeed, African–American patients are less responsive to monotherapy with ACE inhibitors, ARBs and β blockers for hypertension than are Caucasian patients. Administration of each of these drugs in a two-drug combination with the diuretic, hydrochlorothiazide (HCTZ), however, produces similar efficacy in African–American and Caucasian patients [12,13]. For example, telmisartan 80 mg combined with HCTZ 12.5 mg is effective and well tolerated in African-American patients with mild-to-moderate hypertension, providing greater antihypertensive activity than do the corresponding monotherapies (Figure 4.1) [12].

As the cardioprotective effects of blockade of the renin–angiotensin system are largely independent of blood pressure, combination therapy provides vascular protection for hypertensive African–American patients without efficacy being compromised. More aggressive use of combination therapy may improve clinical outcomes among high-risk, hypertensive African–Americans. According to guidelines from the International Society of Hypertension on Blacks, many African–Americans with hypertension will require combination therapy as first-line therapy to enable them to reach appropriate blood pressure goals [8,14].

Patients with diabetes

The incidence of hypertension in patients with diabetes is approximately two-fold higher than in age-matched subjects without the disease and, conversely, individuals with hypertension are at increased risk of developing diabetes compared with normotensive individuals [15]. Up to 75% of cases of cardiovascular disease in patients with diabetes can be attributed to hypertension; therefore, aggressive management of elevated blood pressure is required to reduce cardiovascular morbidity and mortality in these patients. Thiazide diuretics, β blockers, ACE inhibitors, ARBs, and calcium channel blockers are indicated for patients with hypertension and type 2 diabetes to reduce cardiovascular and renal risk; however, most of these patients will need at least two antihypertensive agents to reach the recommended goal of less than 130/80 mmHg, and combination therapy may be beneficial [16–18]. Antihypertensive drugs can significantly influence the probability that otherwise healthy individuals will develop metabolic

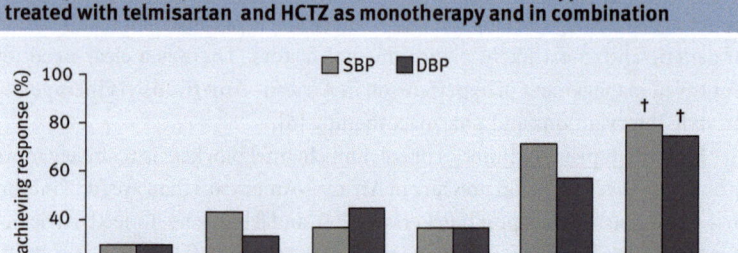

Figure 4.1 Blood pressure response rates in African–Americans with hypertension treated with telmisartan and HCTZ as monotherapy and in combination. SBP response defined as >10 mmHg reduction from baseline in supine SBP; DBP response defined as supine DBP <90 mmHg and/or a >10 mmHg reduction from baseline. DBP, diastolic blood pressure; HCTZ, hydrochlorothiazide; SBP, systolic blood pressure; T, telmisartan. Reproduced with permission from McGill JB, Reilly PA. Combination treatment with telmisartan and hydrochlorothiazide in black patients with mild to moderate hypertension. Clin Cardiol 2001; 24(1):66–72.

syndrome or type 2 diabetes [17]. Diuretics and β blockers have a prodiabetic effect, whereas ACE inhibitors and ARBs may prevent diabetes more effectively than the metabolically neutral calcium channel blockers [17].

Combination therapy with a calcium channel blocker (amlodipine) and an ACE inhibitor (fosinopril) has been shown to provide blood pressure control in hypertensive patients with diabetes who were not controlled with monotherapy [19]. Also, the combined use of a calcium channel blocker (diltiazem) and an ACE inhibitor (captopril) in hypertensive patients with diabetic nephropathy has been shown to cause greater blood pressure reduction and have a superior renoprotective effect, with greater reductions in proteinuria, than either agent alone [20]. The combination of low doses of ACE inhibitor and ARB has been shown to have effects similar to those of high-dose ARB in retarding diabetic nephropathy in hypertensive patients with type 2 diabetes [21].

The combination of an ARB with the diuretic HCTZ in the treatment of hypertensive patients with type 2 diabetes has been assessed in several studies. For example, olmesartan–HCTZ has been shown to be effective in reducing blood pressure in elderly hypertensive diabetic patients [22]; and telmisartan–HCTZ has been shown to provide significantly greater blood pressure lowering than valsartan–HCTZ in high-risk, overweight/obese hypertensive patients with diabetes [23]. In a further study, initial combination therapy with losartan–HCTZ has been shown to be more effective than ACE inhibitor (ramipril) monotherapy in achieving blood pressure goals in hypertensive patients with diabetes, with no significant differences in the incidence of adverse experiences [24].

The combined use of an ACE inhibitor (enalapril) with HCTZ in hypertensive patients with type 1 or 2 diabetes has been shown to clearly reduce diastolic blood pressure compared with ACE inhibitor monotherapy, and to be well tolerated [25]. Combined therapy with enalapril–HCTZ has also been shown to significantly reduce blood pressure and albuminuria in hypertensive patients with type 2 diabetes and albuminuria [26]. Also, the addition of HCTZ to fosinopril therapy has been shown to be associated with a metabolic profile similar, or for certain parameters, superior, to that with fosinopril–indapamide therapy in hypertensive patients with diabetes [21].

Patients with metabolic syndrome

Metabolic syndrome (also known as cardiometabolic syndrome or cardiovascular dysmetabolic syndrome) is a cluster of cardiovascular risk factors that identifies individuals at a relatively high, long-term risk for type 2 diabetes and concomitant increased potential for cardiovascular morbidity and mortality [28,29]. The metabolic syndrome is characterized by obesity (particularly central obesity), insulin resistance, impaired glucose tolerance, hypertension, and dyslipidemia (hypertriglyceridemia and low levels of high-density lipoprotein [HDL]-cholesterol). The major risk factors leading to this syndrome are physical inactivity and an atherogenic diet [30,31].

The worldwide prevalence of obesity, insulin resistance, diabetes, dyslipidemia, and hypertension is increasing, which leads to increasing rates of cardiovascular morbidity and mortality. Almost 25% of the adult population in Europe and the USA appear to have metabolic syndrome, with the condition more prevalent in men than in women in recent years [28]. Prevalence of the syndrome is increasing, however, and the increase seems to be steeper in women [28]. The goals of treatment of metabolic syndrome are to prevent cardiovascular disease by altering the risk factors that are components of the syndrome, and to apply lifestyle modifications, including caloric restriction and exercise [28].

For patients with metabolic syndrome, pharmacological treatment is usually necessary to improve blood pressure and lipid profiles, thereby decreasing the risk of cardiovascular disease. Administration of antihypertensive agents as part of a multi-drug approach may decrease the progression of pre-hypertension to hypertension in these patients. Furthermore, blocking the renin–angiotensin system (with ACE inhibitors and ARBs) may prevent new-onset diabetes in patients with metabolic syndrome [17,32,33]. Thus low-dose combination therapy with an ACE inhibitor or ARB and a complementary antihypertensive agent may provide significant benefits to patients with metabolic syndrome in terms of blood pressure reduction and prevention of new-onset diabetes, with minimal side effects. In this respect, significant improvement in blood pressure and metabolic risk factors has been shown with the ARB, irbesartan, in patients with metabolic syndrome; however, there was no evidence of a difference between irbesartan monotherapy and irbesartan–HCTZ combination therapy with regard to the cardiovascular risk profile [34].

Patients with coronary artery disease

The prevention of coronary artery disease is one of the main goals of anti-hypertensive therapy; however, patients who are diagnosed with hypertension often present with associated coronary artery disease at the time of diagnosis [35]. Coronary artery disease in hypertensive patients is a complex and multifactorial process involving not only hemodynamic, neurohormonal and metabolic factors, but also hypertension-induced myocardial and vascular structural changes, which appear to contribute independently to risk for coronary artery disease [35]. Despite clear guidelines and an array of available antihypertensive medications, patients with hypertension and coronary artery disease are often inadequately treated [36]. For these patients, combination therapy with, for example, ACE inhibitors and calcium channel blockers is a more effective strategy than monotherapy and most of them will require it to achieve a target blood pressure of less than 120/80 mmHg [35,37]. They will usually also require a diuretic.

References

1. Nash DT. Systolic hypertension. Geriatrics 2006; 61(12):22–8.
2. Sadowski AV, Redeker NS. The hypertensive elder: a review for the primary care provider. Nurse Pract 1996; 21(5):99–102, 105–12, 118.
3. Papademetriou V. Hypertension and cognitive function. Blood pressure regulation and cognitive function: a review of the literature. Geriatrics 2005; 60(1):20–2, 24.
4. Neutel JM, Weber MA, Julius S, et al. Clinical experience with perindopril in elderly hypertensive patients: a subgroup analysis of a large community trial. Am J Cardiovasc Drugs 2004; 4(5):335–41.
5. Chalmers J, Castaigne A, Morgan T, Chastang C. Long-term efficacy of a new, fixed, very-low-dose angiotensin-converting enzyme-inhibitor/diuretic combination as first-line therapy in elderly hypertensive patients. J Hypertens 2000; 18(3):327–37.
6. Ferdinand KC, Saunders E. Hypertension-related morbidity and mortality in African Americans – why we need to do better. J Clin Hypertens 2006; 8(1 Suppl 1):21–30.

7. Saunders E. Managing hypertension in African-American patients. J Clin Hypertens 2004; 6(4 Suppl 1):19–25.

8. Ferdinand KC, Armani AM. The management of hypertension in African Americans. Crit Pathol Cardiol 2007; 6(2):67–71.

9. Wright JT Jr, Douglas J. Optimal treatment of hypertension and cardiovascular risk reduction in African Americans: treatment approaches for outpatients. J Clin Hypertens 2003; 5(1 Suppl 1):18–25.

10. Saunders E. Tailoring treatment to minority patients. Am J Med 1990; 88(3B):21–23S.

11. Lackland DT, Lin Y, Tilley BC, Egan BM. An assessment of racial differences in clinical practices for hypertension at primary care sites for medically underserved patients. J Clin Hypertens 2004; 6(1):26–31; quiz 32–3.

12. McGill JB, Reilly PA. Combination treatment with telmisartan and hydrochlorothiazide in black patients with mild to moderate hypertension. Clin Cardiol 2001; 24(1):66–72.

13. Bakris GL, Smith DH, Giles TD, White WB, Davidai G, Weber MA. Comparative antihypertensive efficacy of angiotensin receptor blocker-based treatment in African-American and white patients. J Clin Hypertens 2005; 7(10):587–95; quiz 596–7.

14. Douglas JG, Bakris GL, Epstein M, et al. Hypertension in African Americans Working Group of the International Society on Hypertension in Blacks. Management of high blood pressure in African Americans: consensus statement of the Hypertension in African Americans Working Group of the International Society on Hypertension in Blacks. Arch Intern Med 2003; 163(5):525–41.

15. Sowers JR. Recommendations for special populations: diabetes mellitus and the metabolic syndrome. Am J Hypertens 2003; 16(11 Pt 2):41S–45S.

16. Mancia G. The association of hypertension and diabetes: prevalence, cardiovascular risk and protection by blood pressure reduction. Acta Diabetol 2005; 42(Suppl 1):S17–25.

17. Ferdinand KC. Management of cardiovascular risk in patients with type 2 diabetes mellitus as a component of the cardiometabolic syndrome. J Cardiometab Syndr 2006; 1(2):133–40.

18. Giunti S, Cooper M. Management strategies for patients with hypertension and diabetes: why combination therapy is critical. J Clin Hypertens 2006; 8(2):108–13.

19. Tatti P, Pahor M, Byington RP, et al. Outcome results of the fosinopril versus amlodipine cardiovascular events randomized trial (FACET) in patients with hypertension and NIDDM. Diabetes Care 1998; 21:597–603.

20. Bakris GL, Weir MR, DeQuattro V, McMahon FG. Effects of an ACE inhibitor/calcium antagonist combination on proteinuria in diabetic nephropathy. Kidney Int 1998; 54:1283–9.

21. Ogawa S, Takeuchi K, Mori T, Nako K, Tsubono Y, Ito S. Effects of monotherapy of temocapril or candesartan with dose increments or combination therapy with both drugs on the suppression of diabetic nephropathy. Hypertens Res 2007; 30(4):325–34.

22. Fogari R, Derosa G, Zoppi A, et al. Effects of manidipine/delapril versus olmesartan/hydrochlorothiazide combination therapy in elderly hypertensive patients with type 2 diabetes mellitus. Hypertens Res 2008; 31:43–50.

23. Sharma AM, Davidson J, Koval S, Lacourcière Y. Telmisartan/hydrochlorothiazide versus valsartan/hydrochlorothiazide in obese hypertensive patients with type 2 diabetes: the SMOOTH study. Cardiovasc Diabetol 2007; 6:28.

24. Fox JC, Leight K, Sutradhar SC, et al. The JNC 7 approach compared to conventional treatment in diabetic patients with hypertension: a double-blind trial of initial monotherapy vs. combination therapy. J Clin Hypertens (Greenwich). 2004; 6(8):437–42; quiz 443–4.

25. Agrawal R, Marx A, Haller H. Efficacy and safety of lercanidipine versus hydrochlorothiazide as add-on to enalapril in diabetic populations with uncontrolled hypertension. J Hypertens 2006; 24(1):185–92.

26. Fernández R, Puig JG, Rodríguez-Pérez JC, Garrido J, Redon J; TRAVEND Study Group. Effect of two antihypertensive combinations on metabolic control in type-2 diabetic hypertensive patients with albuminuria: a randomised, double-blind study. J Hum Hypertens 2001; 15:849–56.

27. Krum H, Skiba M, Gilbert RE. Comparative metabolic effects of hydrochlorothiazide and indapamide in hypertensive diabetic patients receiving ACE inhibitor therapy. Diabet Med 2003 ;20:708–12.

28. Mitrakou A. Women's health and the metabolic syndrome. Ann NY Acad Sci 2006; 1092:33–48.

29. Darsow T, Kendall D, Maggs D. Is the metabolic syndrome a real clinical entity and should it receive drug treatment? Curr Diab Rep 2006; 6(5):357–64.

30. Deedwania PC, Gupta R. Management issues in the metabolic syndrome. J Assoc Physicians India 2006; 54:797–810.

31. Ganne S, Arora S, Karam J, McFarlane SI. Therapeutic interventions for hypertension in metabolic syndrome: a comprehensive approach. Expert Rev Cardiovasc Ther 2007; 5(2):201–11.

32. Bakris G, Molitch M, Hewkin A, et al., STAR Investigators. Differences in glucose tolerance between fixed-dose antihypertensive drug combinations in people with metabolic syndrome. Diabetes Care 2006; 29(12):2592–7.

33. Nash DT. Rationale for combination therapy in hypertension management: focus on angiotensin receptor blockers and thiazide diuretics. South Med J 2007; 100(4):386–92.

34. Kintscher U, Bramlage P, Paar WD, Thoenes M, Unger T. Irbesartan for the treatment of hypertension in patients with the metabolic syndrome: a sub analysis of the Treat to Target post authorization survey. Prospective observational, two armed study in 14,200 patients. Cardiovasc Diabetol 2007; 6:12.

35. Morisco C, Lembo G, Sarno D, et al. Benefits of combination therapy in hypertensive patients with associated coronary artery disease: a subgroup with specific demands. J Cardiovasc Pharmacol 1998; 31(Suppl 2):S27–33.

36. Docherty A, Dunn FG. Treatment of hypertensive patients with coexisting coronary arterial disease. Curr Opin Cardiol 2003; 18(4):268–71.

37. Elliott WJ, Hewkin AC, Kupfer S, Cooper-DeHoff R, Pepine CJ. A drug dose model for predicting clinical outcomes in hypertensive coronary disease patients. J Clin Hypertens 2005; 7(11):654–63.

Chapter 5

The evidence base for combination therapy

Many clinical studies have shown that treating elevated systolic blood pressure results in a significant reduction in cardiovascular morbidity and mortality; however, multiple drug therapy is required in the majority of patients to achieve the current goals for blood pressure control (see Chapter 1). The use of combination therapy may result in greater decreases in systolic blood pressure, a higher rate of control of blood pressure, and a better adverse event profile than do component monotherapies at the same or higher doses. Studies such as ALLHAT, ASCOT, LIFE and UK PDS demonstrated that combination therapy is superior to monotherapy. The vast majority of outcome studies are of combination therapy as it is unethical to leave patients inadequately treated. Only two outcome studies, FACET and PROGRESS, were set up specifically to test combination versus monotherapy, and in both of these combination therapy was proved superior (see pp. 63–64 and 54–56, respectively). This section summarizes a selection of studies that have been conducted to assess the efficacy and safety of different combination therapies for the treatment of hypertension.

Studies assessing angiotensin II receptor blockers alone and in combination with diuretics

The clinical use of angiotensin II receptor blockers (ARBs) in drug combination therapy is increasing because treatment guidelines now recommend that they should be used not only as second-line therapy but also for treatment-naïve patients whose systolic/diastolic blood pressure is 20/10 mmHg above the target [1,2]. Furthermore, continuation of initial treatment is reported to be higher with ARBs than for any other class of antihypertensive drug [3]. The greater therapeutic compliance with ARBs compared with other types of antihypertensive drug is illustrated in Figure 5.1 [4]. This chapter describes a selection of studies that have been conducted to assess the efficacy and safety of ARBs alone and in combination with diuretics.

J. M. Neutel, *Combination Therapy in Hypertension*,
DOI: 10.1007/978-1-908517-28-9_5, © Springer Healthcare 2011

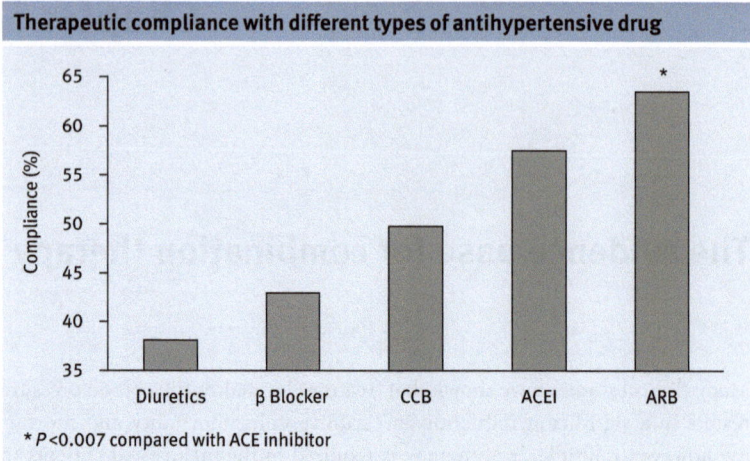

Figure 5.1 Therapeutic compliance with different types of antihypertensive drug.
ACEI, angiotensin-converting enzyme inhibitor; ARB, angiotensin II receptor blocker;
CCB, calcium channel blocker.

Open-label study assessing irbesartan–HCTZ fixed combinations in a sequential treatment regimen (INCLUSIVE study)

The Irbesartan/Hydrochlorothiazide (HCTZ) Blood Pressure Reductions in Diverse Patient Populations (INCLUSIVE) study assessed the efficacy and safety of fixed combinations of irbesartan and HCTZ in a sequential treatment regimen [5]. This was a multicenter, prospective, open-label, single-arm study comprising 1005 patients aged at least 18 years, with uncontrolled systolic blood pressure (140–159 mmHg; 130–159 mmHg for patients with type 2 diabetes mellitus) after at least 4 weeks of antihypertensive monotherapy. Treatment was sequential, as follows: placebo (4–5 weeks); HCTZ 12.5 mg (2 weeks); irbesartan 150 mg–HCTZ 12.5 mg (8 weeks); and irbesartan 300 mg–HCTZ 25 mg (8 weeks). The mean change in systolic blood pressure from baseline (end of placebo phase) to the primary endpoint, week 18 (intent-to-treat population, n=736), was −21.5 mmHg (P <0.001), and the mean change in diastolic blood pressure was −10.4 mmHg (P <0.001). The mean week 18 systolic/diastolic blood pressure was 132.9/81.1 mmHg. Overall, 77% of patients achieved the systolic blood pressure goal (<140 mmHg; <130 mmHg for type 2 diabetes mellitus); 83% achieved the diastolic blood pressure goal (<90 mmHg; <80 mmHg for type 2 diabetes mellitus); and 69% achieved the dual systolic/diastolic blood pressure goal. Treatments were well tolerated. In this study, more than three-quarters of patients whose hypertension was not controlled on monotherapy achieved systolic blood pressure goals with irbesartan–HCTZ combination therapy [5].

Subgroup analysis of the data from the INCLUSIVE study was conducted to assess the effects of irbesartan–HCTZ combination therapy in patients with type 2 diabetes mellitus or metabolic syndrome [6]. In patients with type 2 diabetes mellitus (n=227), the mean change in systolic blood pressure from baseline to week 18 was −18.2 mmHg (P <0.001) and in diastolic blood pressure was −8.7 mmHg (P <0.001). In patients with metabolic syndrome (n=345), the corresponding results were −21.0 mmHg and −10.4 mmHg, respectively (P <0.001). Overall, 56% of diabetic patients and 73% of patients with metabolic syndrome achieved the systolic blood pressure goal (see definition above) [6].

Data from the INCLUSIVE trial were further analyzed to assess the effects of irbesartan–HCTZ combination therapy in different racial/ethnic subgroups [7]. Overall, 515 Caucasians, 191 African–Americans and 119 Hispanics/Latinos who completed the placebo phase were enrolled. The mean change in systolic blood pressure from baseline to week 18 was −21.5 mmHg for Caucasians; −20.7 mmHg for African–Americans and −22.9 mmHg for Hispanics/Latinos (P <0.001 for each). Mean diastolic blood pressure changes were statistically significant (P <0.001) and similar among racial/ethnic subgroups. By week 18, 70% of Caucasians, 66% of African–Americans, and 65% of Hispanics/Latinos achieved the dual systolic/diastolic blood pressure goal (see definition above).

Double-blind study comparing irbesartan–HCTZ combination therapy and irbesartan monotherapy in severe hypertension

A randomized, double-blind, actively controlled study was conducted to compare the efficacy and safety of once-daily irbesartan–HCTZ combination therapy with irbesartan monotherapy in patients with severe hypertension [8]. Untreated patients and patients who were not controlled on monotherapy (seated diastolic blood pressure ≥110 mmHg) received fixed-dose irbesartan 150 mg–HCTZ 12.5 mg combination therapy for 7 weeks, force titrated to irbesartan 300 mg–HCTZ 25 mg at week 1 (n=468), or irbesartan 150 mg monotherapy, force titrated to 300 mg at week 1 (n=269). The primary endpoint was seated diastolic blood pressure of less than 90 mmHg at week 5. The primary endpoint was achieved by significantly more patients on combination therapy compared with on monotherapy (47.2% compared with 33.2%; P=0.0005). Also, significantly more patients achieved systolic/diastolic blood pressure of less than 140/90 mmHg at week 5 on combination therapy compared with on monotherapy (34.6% compared with 19.2%; P <0.0001). Greater and more rapid blood pressure reduction was achieved with irbesartan–HCTZ combination therapy compared with irbesartan monotherapy, without additional side effects [8].

Double-blind study comparing irbesartan–HCTZ combination therapy and irbesartan monotherapy in moderate hypertension

A randomized, double-blind, parallel-group study was conducted to compare the efficacy and safety of irbesartan–HCTZ combination therapy with irbesartan and HCTZ monotherapy in patients with moderate hypertension (defined as seated systolic blood pressure 160–179 mmHg when seated diastolic blood pressure <110 mmHg; or seated diastolic blood pressure 100–109 mmHg when seated systolic blood pressure <180 mmHg) [9].

Patients were randomized 3:1:1 to treatment with irbesartan 300 mg–HCTZ 25 mg combination therapy (n=328), irbesartan 300 mg monotherapy (n=106), or HCTZ monotherapy 25 mg (n=104). Treatment was initiated at half dose, force titrated to full dose after 2 weeks, and then full dose was administered for a further 10 weeks. The primary efficacy variable was the mean reduction in seated systolic blood pressure from baseline to week 8. The mean reduction in seated systolic blood pressure from baseline to week 8 with irbesartan–HCTZ combination therapy (27.1 mmHg) was significantly greater than with irbesartan monotherapy (22.1 mmHg; P <0.05) or HCTZ monotherapy (15.7 mmHg; P <0.0001), as was the mean reduction in seated diastolic blood pressure (14.6 versus 11.6 and 7.3 mmHg, respectively, P <0.005 for both comparisons). Irbesartan–HCTZ combination therapy was associated with the greatest rate of decline and total degree of decline in seated systolic blood pressure, and HCTZ with the least. Furthermore, a significantly greater percentage of patients reached a treatment goal of seated systolic/diastolic blood pressure <140/90 mmHg by week 8 on irbesartan–HCTZ combination therapy (53.4%) than on irbesartan monotherapy (40.6%; P <0.05) or HCTZ monotherapy (20.2%; P <0.0001), and this difference continued (55.8% compared with 34 and 25%, respectively, at week 12; P <0.0001 for both comparisons).

In this study, rapid and sustained reductions in both systolic and diastolic blood pressures were shown with irbesartan–HCTZ combination therapy in patients with moderate hypertension, and the treatment was well tolerated.

Open-label extension study assessing telmisartan alone or with HCTZ and/or other antihypertensives using a fixed-titration regimen

An open-label, multicenter, extension study was conducted to assess the efficacy and tolerability of telmisartan 80 mg administered alone or with HCTZ and/or other antihypertensive agents over a maximal 1-year treatment period [10]. This was an extension of a 6-week randomized study that compared telmisartan 80 mg with losartan 50 mg–HCTZ 12.5 mg combination therapy in patients with mild-to-moderate hypertension.

Of the 690 patients who completed the 6-week study, 489 patients (70.9%) continued in the extension study. A fixed-titration regimen was used: all patients initially received telmisartan 80 mg, with the stepwise addition of HCTZ 12.5 mg, HCTZ 25 mg, and/or other antihypertensives to attain diastolic blood pressure control (<90 mmHg). At the final visit, diastolic blood pressure control was achieved in 70.0% of patients who were maximally titrated to telmisartan 80 mg, 55.8% titrated to telmisartan 80 mg–HCTZ 12.5 mg, 54.7% titrated to telmisartan 80 mg–HCTZ 25 mg, and 64.7% titrated to telmisartan 80 mg plus another antihypertensive with or without HCTZ (12.5 or 25 mg). The reductions in diastolic and systolic blood pressure observed in the preceding randomized trial continued during extension treatment. Progressively greater blood pressure reductions occurred with the sequential addition of HCTZ and other antihypertensives. Adding HCTZ 12.5 mg to telmisartan 80 mg was particularly effective in enhancing antihypertensive efficacy. All treatments were well tolerated.

This extension study showed that telmisartan 80 mg administered alone or with HCTZ (12.5 or 25 mg) and/or other antihypertensives maintains a clinically significant therapeutic effect over the long term in patients with mild-to-moderate hypertension [10].

Community-based study assessing telmisartan–HCTZ combination therapy and telmisartan monotherapy (MICCAT-2)

A large practice-based study was conducted to evaluate the effects of telmisartan alone and in combination with HCTZ on 24-hour blood pressure profiles, including the early morning period, which is associated with high cardiovascular risk [11]. Patients with hypertension who were either untreated or currently on treatment were started on, or switched to, telmisartan 40 mg/day. Patients whose blood pressure was still at least 140/85 mmHg after 2 weeks had the dose of telmisartan increased to 80 mg/day and, if necessary, HCTZ 12.5 mg was added after a further 4 weeks and continued for a final 4-week period. Baseline and end-of-treatment 24-hour ambulatory blood pressure monitoring measurements were completed in 1619 patients.

There were highly significant reductions in both the daytime (–11.8/–7.2 mmHg) and the night-time (–9.6/–5.7 mmHg) mean blood pressure following telmisartan alone or in combination with HCTZ. The 24-hour profiles showed evidence for sustained pharmacodynamic effects of telmisartan over the entire dosing period.

Early morning (post-awakening) blood pressure decreased by −11.5/−7.0 mmHg ($P<0.001$) in the entire study cohort (reductions were similar with monotherapy and combination therapy) and by −17.2/−10.1 mmHg in patients with large morning blood pressure surges (>30 mmHg change in systolic blood pressure).

In this community-based study, telmisartan-based therapy induced highly significant reductions in systolic and diastolic blood pressure over 24 hours and was particularly effective in reducing blood pressure during the early morning period.

Study comparing low-dose losartan–HCTZ combination therapy and stepped-care therapy

Patients with stage 2 or 3 hypertension and a mean daytime systolic ambulatory blood pressure of at least 135 mmHg were enrolled into a study to investigate whether initiating therapy with a combination of losartan and HCTZ enables faster blood pressure control and fewer medications than the usual stepped-care approach [12]. Patients were randomly assigned to receive losartan 50 mg–HCTZ 12.5 mg titrated to losartan 100 mg–HCTZ 25 mg, or HCTZ 12.5 mg–atenolol 50 mg. Amlodipine 5 mg was then added, if needed, to achieve a daytime systolic blood pressure of less than 130 mmHg (primary endpoint).

The primary endpoint was achieved by significantly more patients who received low-dose losartan–HCTZ combination therapy than by those who received stepped-care therapy (63.5% compared with 37.5%; $P=0.008$). Initial therapy with losartan–HCTZ was associated with significantly greater decreases in ambulatory blood pressure during each 24-hour period after 6 weeks of therapy. Also, the primary endpoint was achieved with no more than two drugs in 30.0% of patients who received combination therapy compared with 14.7% of patients who received stepped-care therapy ($P=0.03$). Tolerability was significantly better in the combination therapy group than in the stepped-care therapy group (incidence of adverse events of 40.0% compared with 65.6%; $P=0.006$).

This study showed that initiating antihypertensive therapy with losartan–HCTZ combination therapy enables target blood pressure to be achieved faster in a higher proportion of patients, with fewer adverse events and less need for a third drug, than the conventional stepped-care approach [12].

Antihypertensive treatment algorithm with olmesartan medoxomil as the initial agent

The effectiveness of an antihypertensive treatment algorithm with the ARB, olmesartan medoxomil, as the initial agent has been studied in a 24-week, open-label study in patients (n=201) with mean seated diastolic blood pressure of 90–109 mmHg [13]. Following placebo run-in, all patients received olmesartan medoxomil 20 mg/day for 4 weeks. At subsequent 4-week intervals, the regimen was modified in patients whose blood pressure remained above 130/85 mmHg: uptitration of olmesartan medoxomil to 40 mg/day; addition of HCTZ 12.5 mg/day; uptitration of HCTZ to 25 mg/day; addition of amlodipine besylate 5 mg/day; and uptitration of amlodipine besylate to 10 mg/day. Patients who achieved a blood pressure of 130/85 mmHg or lower left the study.

At week 24, reductions in blood pressure from baseline were 33.7/18.2 mmHg. Altogether, 87.7% of patients reached the goal blood pressure of 130/85 mmHg or lower and 93.3% achieved a blood pressure of 140/90 mmHg or lower. In this study, an antihypertensive algorithm with olmesartan medoxomil as the initial agent controlled blood pressure in the majority of patients, but more than 60% of patients also required the use of a thiazide diuretic or a thiazide and a calcium channel blocker [13].

Dose-titration study assessing olmesartan medoxomil with or without HCTZ

An aggressive treatment program for stage 2 systolic hypertension (pretreatment systolic blood pressure ≥160 mmHg) using olmesartan medoxomil and HCTZ was investigated in an open-label, dose-titration study [14]. A total of 170 patients received olmesartan medoxomil 20 mg/day for 3 weeks. Patients whose seated systolic/diastolic blood pressure remained at least 120/80 mmHg were advanced to successive 3-week courses of olmesartan medoxomil 40 mg/day, olmesartan medoxomil 40 mg/day–HCTZ 12.5 mg/day, and olmesartan medoxomil 40 mg/day–HCTZ 25 mg/day. The initial dose of olmesartan medoxomil (20 mg/day) reduced mean systolic blood pressure by 16.9 mmHg (P <0.001), and there were further dose-dependent decreases in mean systolic blood pressure to a maximum of 34.7 mmHg with olmesartan medoxomil 40 mg/day–HCTZ 25 mg/day (Figure 5.2). At the end of the study, 75% of patients achieved the target systolic blood pressure (<140 mmHg) and 16% achieved normalization of systolic blood pressure (<120 mmHg) (Figure 5.2). Treatment was well tolerated at all doses. This study showed that an olmesartan medoxomil-based regimen, with or without HCTZ in conventional doses, is effective in controlling and normalizing blood pressure in patients with stage 2 systolic hypertension.

All patients whose blood pressure remained above 120/80 mmHg (n=105) on olmesartan medoxomil 40 mg/day–HCTZ 25 mg/day at the end of the 12-week

Changes in blood pressure after treatment with olmesartan medoxomil with or without hydrochlorothiazide				
Week	3	6	9	12	16 (extension)
Treatment step	O 20 mg	O 40 mg	O 40 mg + H 12.5 mg	O 40 mg + H 25 mg	O 40 mg + H 50 mg
	(n=169)	(n=160)	(n=157)	(n=144)	(n=106)
Mean change in SBP (mmHg)	−16.9	−18.4	−30.3	−34.7	−38.3
SBP <140 mmHg (%)	17.8	30.8	58.0	75.1	81.1
SBP/DBP <140/90 mmHg (%)	15.4	29.0	55.6	70.4	77.5
SBP <120 mmHg (%)	1.2	1.2	6.5	16.0	27.8
SBP/DBP <120/80 mmHg (%)	1.2	1.2	5.9	15.4	27.2

Figure 5.2 **Changes in blood pressure after treatment with olmesartan medoxomil with or without hydrochlorothiazide.** DBP, diastolic blood pressure; H, hydrochlorothiazide; O, olmesartan; SBP, systolic blood pressure. Reproduced with permission from Izzo J, Neutel J, Dubiel R, Walker F. P-158. Efficacy of olmesartan medoxomil (O) and O/hydrochlorothiazide (H) in achieving blood pressure (BP) control and normalization in stage 2 systolic hypertension (HTN). Am J Hypertens 2005; 18 (5 Pt 2): 64A.

study were included in an extension phase, in which they received olmesartan medoxomil 40 mg/day–HCTZ 50 mg/day for 4 weeks [14]. Increasing HCTZ from 25 mg/day to 50 mg/day decreased systolic blood pressure by 3.6 mmHg, increased rates of blood pressure control (<140/90 mmHg) from 70.4 to 77.5%, and increased rates of blood pressure normalization (<120/80 mmHg) from 15.4 to 27.2% (Figure 5.2). The combination was well tolerated. Olmesartan medoxomil 40 mg/day–HCTZ 50 mg/day is, therefore, a potentially effective strategy for managing stage 2 systolic hypertension [15]. Olmesartan medoxomil may also have end-organ protective effects that provide additional clinical benefit [3].

The metabolic consequences of combination therapy with olmesartan medoxomil and HCTZ were also assessed in the study [16]. Serum potassium, glucose, and uric acid levels remained within normal limits for all olmesartan medoxomil–HCTZ combinations used in the study. There were similar small changes in glucose and uric acid across all HCTZ doses, while serum potassium did not change (Figure 5.3). The addition of HCTZ to olmesartan medoxomil does not, therefore, cause significant metabolic disturbance across the HCTZ dosing range from 12.5 mg daily to 50 mg daily.

Metabolic effects of combination therapy with olmesartan medoxomil and hydrochlorothiazide

Metabolic variable, mean (n)	Olmesartan medoxomil–hydrochlorothiazide (mg/day)			
	Baseline	40–12.5	40–25	40–50
K⁺ (mmol/L)	4.29 (164)	4.30 (151)	4.28 (137)	4.23 (88)
Glucose (mg/dL)	104 (165)	108 (150)	109 (140)	110 (88)
Uric acid (mg/dL)	6.03 (166)	6.95 (151)	7.41 (141)	7.57 (89)

Figure 5.3 Metabolic effects of combination therapy with olmesartan medoxomil and hydrochlorothiazide. Reproduced with permission from Izzo J, Neutel J, Dubiel R, Walker F. P-159. Metabolic effects and safety of hydrochlorothiazide (HCTZ) in combination with olmesartan medoxomil (OLM) in stage 2 systolic hypertension (HTN). Am J Hypertens 2005; 18 (5 Pt 2): 64A.

Studies assessing an angiotensin-converting enzyme inhibitor in combination with a diuretic

Combination therapy with angiotensin-converting enzyme (ACE) inhibitors and thiazide diuretics has been advocated for many years [17]. These drugs in combination have been shown to improve blood pressure reduction over either drug used alone, to be effective in a wide range of patient populations, and to be accompanied by fewer adverse metabolic effects than the thiazides alone [17]. Two studies are described below. One study compared low-dose ACE inhibitor–thiazide diuretic combination therapy with other strategies in the treatment of hypertension, and the other study assessed ACE inhibitor-based therapy with discretionary addition of diuretic in hypertensive and non-hypertensive patients with a history of cerebrovascular disease.

Study comparing low-dose combination therapy, sequential monotherapy and stepped-care therapy (STRATHE study)

The efficacy and tolerability of three different strategies in the treatment of hypertension – low-dose combination therapy, sequential monotherapy, and stepped-care therapy – were compared in a randomized study comprising patients with uncomplicated essential hypertension (Strategies of Treatment in Hypertension: Evaluation; STRATHE study) [18]. Patients in the low-dose combination group (n=180) initially received a preparation containing the ACE inhibitor, perindopril (2 mg), and the diuretic, indapamide (0.625 mg), with the possibility of increasing the doses in two steps to 4 mg and 1.25 mg, respectively. Patients in the sequential monotherapy group (n=176) initially received atenolol 50 mg, which was replaced, if necessary, by losartan 50 mg, and then by amlodipine 5 mg. Patients in the stepped-care therapy group (n=177) initially received valsartan 40 mg, then valsartan 80 mg, then, if needed, valsartan 80 mg co-administered with HCTZ 12.5 mg.

In this study, the percentage of patients who achieved target blood pressure (<140/90 mmHg) was significantly higher with low-dose combination therapy (62%) compared with sequential monotherapy (49%, $P=0.02$) and stepped-care therapy (47%, $P=0.005$). The percentage of patients who achieved normalization of blood pressure without experiencing drug-related adverse events was also significantly higher with low-dose combination therapy (56%) compared with sequential monotherapy (42%, $P=0.002$) and stepped-care therapy (42%, $P=0.004$).

Study assessing angiotensin-converting enzyme inhibitor-based therapy with discretionary addition of diuretic (PROGRESS study)

The effects of an ACE inhibitor (perindopril) based blood pressure-lowering regimen on major cardiac events among hypertensive and non-hypertensive patients with a history of cerebrovascular disease were assessed in the randomized, double-blind, Perindopril Protection Against Recurrent Stroke Study (PROGRESS) [19]. A total of 6105 patients with a history of stroke or transient ischemic attack were randomly assigned to receive active treatment (n=3051) or placebo (n=3054). Active treatment comprised perindopril 4 mg/day, with the addition of the diuretic indapamide (2.5 mg/day, or 2 mg/day in Japan) at the discretion of the treating physicians (indapamide was added for patients with neither an indication for, nor a contraindication to, a diuretic).

During a mean follow-up period of 3.9 years, active treatment reduced blood pressure by 9/4 mmHg compared with placebo and decreased the occurrence of stroke (the primary outcome) by 28%. Active treatment also reduced the risk of major coronary events by 26% (95% CI: 6–42%; $P=0.02$) and the risk of congestive heart failure by 26% (5–42%; $P=0.02$) – see Figure 5.4A and B, respectively. For each of these outcomes, there was no clear evidence of differences between the treatment effects in patients classified as hypertensive or non-hypertensive, and those with or without a history of coronary heart disease. These results indicate that among patients with cerebrovascular disease, blood pressure lowering with a regimen involving perindopril and indapamide not only reduced the risk of stroke, but also substantially reduced the risks of cardiac outcomes.

The effects of a perindopril-based blood pressure-lowering regimen on the risk of recurrent stroke according to stroke subtype and medical history among hypertensive and non-hypertensive patients with a history of cerebrovascular disease were also assessed in PROGRESS [20]. During the mean follow-up period of 3.9 years, active treatment reduced the absolute rates of ischemic stroke from 10% to 8% (relative risk reduction [RRR] 24%;

Effect of perindopril alone and in combination with indapamide in the PROGRESS study

A. Major coronary events[a]

	No. of events/total participants		Favors active	Favors placebo	Risk reduction, % (95% CI)
	Active	Placebo			
Effects in all participants					
Total major coronary events	115/3051	154/3054			26 (6 to 42)
Effects in subgroups					
Combination therapy	67/1770	102/1774			35 (12 to 52)
Single drug therapy	48/1281	52/1280			7 (−37 to 38)
Hypertensive	62/1464	81/1452			20 (−12 to 43)
Not hypertensive	53/1587	73/1602			27 (−4 to 49)
CHD at baseline	40/493	53/490			24 (−15 to 50)
No CHD at baseline	75/2558	101/2564			26 (0 to 45)

0.5   1.0   2.0
Hazard ratio

B. Cerebrovascular events[b]

	No. of events/total participants		Favors active	Favors placebo	Risk reduction, % (95% CI)
	Active	Placebo			
Effects in all participants					
Total congestive heart failure	113/3051	151/3054			26 (5 to 42)
Effects in subgroups					
Combination therapy	55/1770	82/1774			34 (7 to 53)
Single drug therapy	58/1281	69/1280			16 (−19 to 41)
Hypertensive	56/1464	75/1452			27 (−3 to 48)
Not hypertensive	57/1587	76/1602			27 (−4 to 49)
CHD at baseline	37/493	59/490			41 (10 to 61)
No CHD at baseline	76/2558	92/2564			18 (−11 to 40)

0.5   1.0   2.0
Hazard ratio

[a]P for homogeneity for all subgroups >0.1.
[b]P for homogeneity for all subgroups >0.2.

Figure 5.4 Effect of perindopril alone and in combination with indapamide in the PROGRESS study. Diamond represents overall effect, with tips at 95% CI. CHD, coronary heart disease. Reproduced with permission from PROGRESS Collaborative Group. Effects of a perindopril-based blood pressure lowering regimen on cardiac outcomes among patients with cerebrovascular disease. Eur Heart J 2003; 24(5):475–84.

95% confidence interval [CI] 10–35) and the absolute rates of intracerebral hemorrhage from 2% to 1% (RRR 50%; 95% CI 26–67). The relative risk of any stroke during follow-up was reduced by 26% (95% CI 12–38) among patients whose baseline cerebrovascular event was an ischemic stroke, and by 49% (95% CI 18–68) among those whose baseline event was an intracerebral hemorrhage [20]. Other drug therapies (antiplatelet therapy or other antihypertensive agents), residual neurological signs, atrial fibrillation, or the time since the last cerebrovascular event did not appear to modify treatment effects [20]. The reduced stroke risk associated with perindopril-based blood pressure-lowering in the patients in this study was consistent across different stroke subtypes and among major clinical subgroups. The results of this study indicate that instigation of an effective blood pressure-lowering regimen may benefit patients with a history of cerebrovascular events and should be routinely considered for such patients.

Studies assessing calcium channel blockers in combination with ACE inhibitors

Fixed-dose compounds that combine a calcium antagonist and an ACE inhibitor are associated with excellent efficacy, safety, and tolerability in hypertensive patients. As calcium channel blockers and ACE inhibitors work through different mechanisms, combining these drug classes may have more beneficial effects on arteries than using these agents singly in high doses. Furthermore, the combination of ACE inhibitors with calcium channel blockers improves the dose-dependent pedal edema associated with calcium antagonist monotherapy. Simultaneous administration of ACE inhibitors and calcium channel blockers has been reported to be particularly effective in the treatment of hypertensive patients with coronary artery disease [21]. Below are described studies that have been conducted to assess the efficacy and safety of combination therapy with calcium channel blockers and ACE inhibitors.

Community-based study comparing amlodipine–benazepril combination therapy and amlodipine monotherapy

Community-based studies are conducted to determine the degree to which therapeutic interventions will succeed in real world settings. A large practice-based clinical study was conducted to compare the blood pressure-lowering efficacy, tolerability, and effect on edema of fixed-dose amlodipine–benazepril combination therapy with those of amlodipine monotherapy in patients with mild-to-moderate hypertension who were currently taking amlodipine [22].

Eligible patients either had inadequate blood pressure control on amlodipine (diastolic blood pressure ≥90 mmHg; group 1; n=6410), or were not tolerating amlodipine (diastolic blood pressure ≤90 mmHg, but with edema; group 2; n=1502). These patients were switched from amlodipine 5 mg or 10 mg to combination therapy with either amlodipine 5 mg–benazepril 10 mg or amlodipine 5 mg–benazepril 20 mg for 4 weeks. The primary efficacy outcome for group 1 was change in mean sitting diastolic blood pressure and that for group 2 was the percentage of patients whose edema improved during amlodipine–benazepril combination therapy compared with amlodipine monotherapy.

In group 1, mean sitting systolic blood pressure was reduced by 15.6 mmHg ($P <0.001$) and mean sitting diastolic blood pressure was reduced by 11.5 mmHg ($P <0.001$) from baseline to week 4 (Figure 5.5). A total of 85% of patients in group 2 who received amlodipine–benazepril combination therapy experienced improvement in edema compared with baseline levels: edema completely resolved in 42% of patients; 43% of patients had improved edema; 13% of patients had no change in edema; and in 2% of patients, edema had worsened (Figure 5.6).

These results show that amlodipine–benazepril fixed-dose combination therapy is safe and effective in the treatment of hypertensive patients who

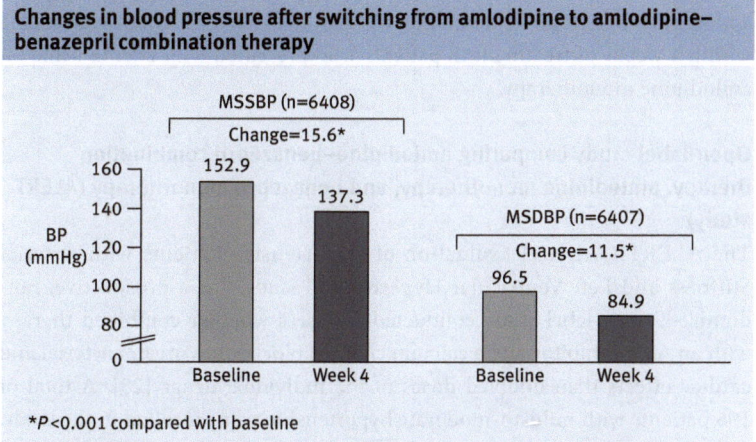

Changes in blood pressure after switching from amlodipine to amlodipine–benazepril combination therapy

*P<0.001 compared with baseline

Figure 5.5 Changes in blood pressure after switching from amlodipine to amlodipine–benazepril combination therapy. Eligible patients had inadequate blood pressure control on amlodipine (diastolic blood pressure ≥90 mmHg; n=6410). BP, blood pressure; MSDBP, mean sitting diastolic blood pressure; MSSBP, mean sitting systolic blood pressure. Reproduced with permission from Messerli FH, Weir MR, Neutel JM. Combination therapy of amlodipine/benazepril versus monotherapy of amlodipine in a practice-based setting. Am J Hypertens 2002; 15(6):550–6.

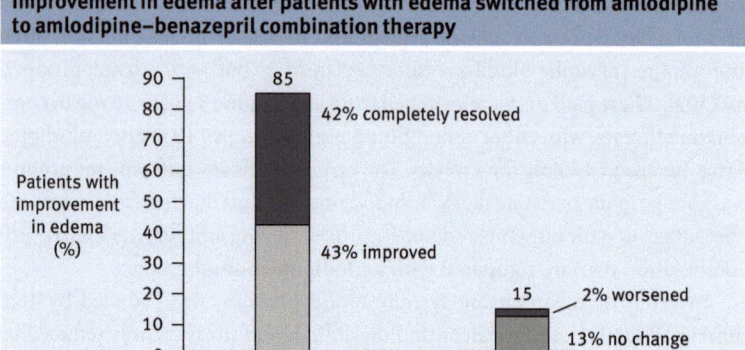

Figure 5.6 Improvement in edema after patients with edema switched from amlodipine to amlodipine–benazepril combination therapy. Patients who were not tolerant of amlodipine (diastolic blood pressure ≤90 mmHg, with edema (n=1502). Improvement in edema was similar for men and women. Reproduced with permission from Messerli FH, Weir MR, Neutel JM. Combination therapy of amlodipine/benazepril versus monotherapy of amlodipine in a practice-based setting. Am J Hypertens 2002; 15(6):550–6.

were either uncontrolled on, or intolerant of, amlodipine monotherapy. The amlodipine–benazepril combination was also associated with improved edema within 4 weeks of treatment in patients who presented with edema while on amlodipine monotherapy.

Open-label study comparing amlodipine–benazepril combination therapy, amlodipine monotherapy, and benazepril monotherapy (ALERT study)

The ALERT (A Lotrel Evaluation of Hypertensive Patients with Arterial Stiffness and Left Ventricular Hypertrophy) study was a prospective, randomized, open-label study conducted to assess whether combined therapy with an ACE inhibitor and a calcium channel blocker has greater arterial and cardiac effects than doubled doses of the individual drugs [23]. A total of 106 patients with mild-to-moderate hypertension were enrolled in the study. Patients were randomized to amlodipine 5 mg or benazepril 20 mg for 2 weeks. After this, depending on randomization assignment, they were force titrated to amlodipine 10 mg or benazepril 40 mg, or to amlodipine 5 mg–benazepril 20 mg combination therapy for 22 weeks. Arterial distensibility was assessed using the DynaPulse ambulatory system, and left ventricular mass was assessed by echocardiography.

There was a statistically significant reduction (P <0.0001) in mean 24-hour systolic blood pressure and mean 24-hour diastolic blood pressure at the end of treatment compared with baseline in all three treatment groups (Figure 5.6). One between-group comparison was statistically significant: the reduction in mean 24-hour systolic blood pressure was statistically significantly greater with combination therapy compared with benazepril alone (P <0.05) (Figure 5.7).

Arterial distensibility was increased more with combination therapy (0.71% ± 0.51% mL/mmHg) than it was with amlodipine monotherapy (0.28% ± 0.69% mL/mmHg; P=0.008) or benazepril monotherapy (0.39% ± 0.62% mL/mmHg; P=0.03) (Figure 5.8).

There was a statistically significantly greater decrease in left ventricular mass with combination treatment (64 ± 56 g) compared with amlodipine (28 ± 47 g; P <0.02); the difference from benazepril (42 ± 50 g) was not

Change in blood pressure in the ALERT study comparing amlodipine–benazepril combination therapy with monotherapy

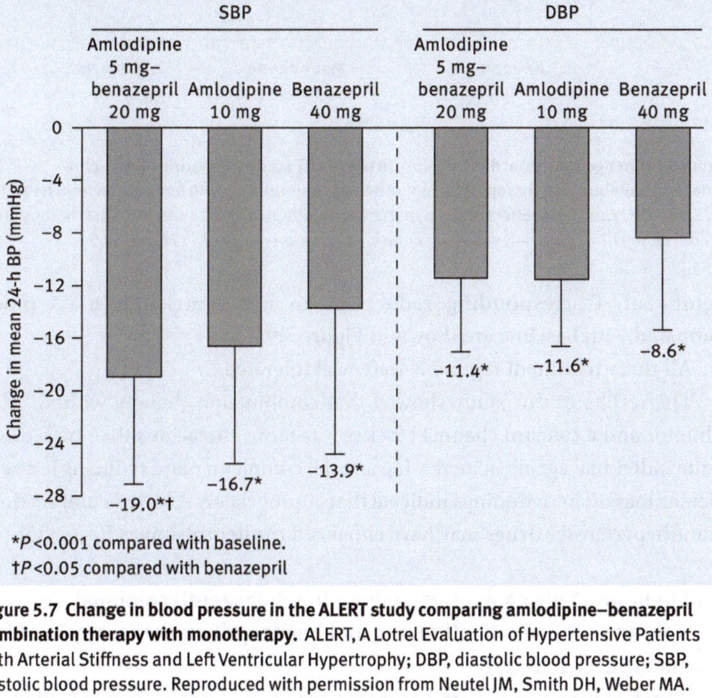

*P<0.001 compared with baseline.
†P<0.05 compared with benazepril

Figure 5.7 Change in blood pressure in the ALERT study comparing amlodipine–benazepril combination therapy with monotherapy. ALERT, A Lotrel Evaluation of Hypertensive Patients with Arterial Stiffness and Left Ventricular Hypertrophy; DBP, diastolic blood pressure; SBP, systolic blood pressure. Reproduced with permission from Neutel JM, Smith DH, Weber MA. Effect of antihypertensive monotherapy and combination therapy on arterial distensibility and left ventricular mass. Am J Hypertens 2004; 17(1):37–42.

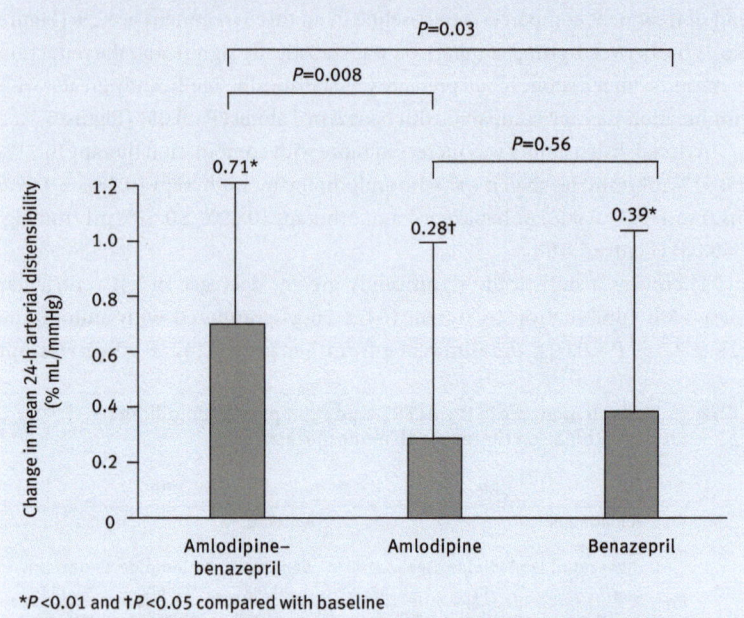

Change in arterial distensibility in the ALERT study comparing amlodipine–benazepril combination therapy with monotherapy

P=0.03

P=0.008

P=0.56

0.71*

0.28†

0.39*

Amlodipine–benazepril

Amlodipine

Benazepril

Change in mean 24-h arterial distensibility (% mL/mmHg)

P<0.01 and †*P*<0.05 compared with baseline

Figure 5.8 Change in arterial distensibility in the ALERT study comparing amlodipine–benazepril combination therapy with monotherapy. Reproduced with permission from Neutel JM, Smith DH, Weber MA. Effect of antihypertensive monotherapy and combination therapy on arterial distensibility and left ventricular mass. Am J Hypertens 2004; 17(1):37–42.

significant. Corresponding reductions in left ventricular mass index compared with baseline are shown in Figure 5.9.

All three treatment regimens were well tolerated.

The results of this study showed that combination therapy with an ACE inhibitor and a calcium channel blocker was more efficacious than high doses of the individual agents in increasing arterial compliance and reducing left ventricular mass. These findings indicate that appropriately selected combinations of antihypertensive drugs may have enhanced cardioprotective effects [23].

Double-blind study comparing amlodipine–benazepril combination therapy, amlodipine monotherapy, and benazepril monotherapy in older patients (SELECT study)

The Systolic Evaluation of Lotrel Efficacy and Comparative Therapies (SELECT) study was a randomized, multicenter, prospective, double-blind, parallel-group

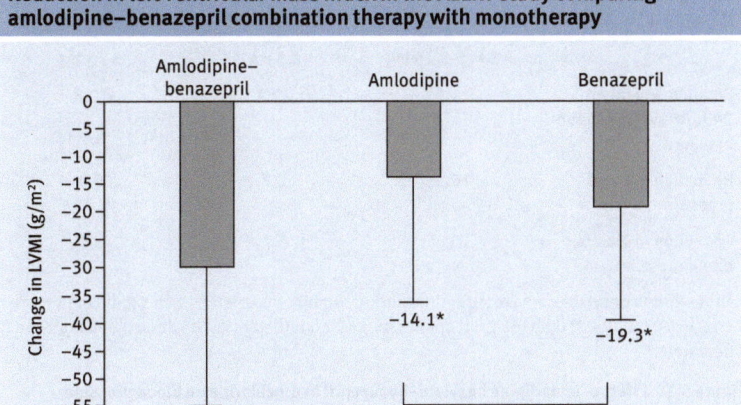

Reduction in left ventricular mass index in the ALERT study comparing amlodipine–benazepril combination therapy with monotherapy

Figure 5.9 Reduction in left ventricular mass index in the ALERT study comparing amlodipine–benazepril combination therapy with monotherapy. LVMI, left ventricular mass index. Reproduced with permission from Neutel JM, Smith DH, Weber MA. Effect of antihypertensive monotherapy and combination therapy on arterial distensibility and left ventricular mass. Am J Hypertens 2004; 17(1):37–42.

study that compared daily treatment with amlodipine besylate 5 mg–benazepril hydrochloride 20 mg combination therapy (n=149), amlodipine besylate 5 mg monotherapy (n=146), and benazepril hydrochloride 20 mg monotherapy (n=148) in patients aged at least 55 years with stage 2 hypertension (systolic blood pressure in the range 160–200 mmHg and diastolic blood pressure in the range 60–100 mmHg) [24,25]. Eligible patients had newly diagnosed hypertension or had discontinued previous antihypertensive medication. Patients received treatment after a 2- to 4-week placebo phase. Twenty-four-hour ambulatory blood pressure monitoring was used to identify patients with systolic hypertension and to determine the impact of 8 weeks of treatment on 24-hour systolic blood pressure, pulse pressure, and diastolic blood pressure.

Amlodipine besylate–benazepril hydrochloride combination therapy was significantly more effective in reducing systolic blood pressure, pulse pressure and diastolic blood pressure than either drug as monotherapy (P <0.0001) (Figure 5.10) [25]. Also, significantly greater percentages of

Effect of amlodipine besylate–benazepril hydrochloride on blood pressure parameters compared with the component drugs alone

	A 5 mg–B 20 mg	A 5 mg	B 20 mg
Reduction in mean 24-hour systolic blood pressure	21.1*	12.4	10.8
Reduction in pulse pressure	10.5*	6.7	5.0
Reduction in diastolic blood pressure	10.6*	5.7	5.7

*Amlodipine besylate–benazepril hydrochloride combination therapy was significantly more effective ($P < 0.0001$) than the component drugs as monotherapy for all three blood pressure parameters.

Figure 5.10 Effect of amlodipine besylate–benazepril hydrochloride on blood pressure parameters compared with the component drugs alone. A, Amlodipine besylate; B benazepril hydrochloride. Data from Neutel JM, Smith DHG, Weber MA, Nwose OM, Schofield L, Gatlin M. P-409. Initial combination therapy in older patients with systolic hypertension: results of the systolic evaluation of lotrel efficacy and comparative therapies (SELECT) study. Am J Hypertens 2004; 17 (5 Pt 2): 183A.

patients achieved blood pressure control (systolic blood pressure <140 mmHg) with combination therapy (65%) compared with either drug as monotherapy (28% for amlodipine besylate; 34% for benazepril hydrochloride; $P < 0.0001$) [25]. Adverse event rates were low in all three treatment groups. The incidence of peripheral edema in patients who received combination therapy was lower than in patients who received amlodipine besylate alone. This study showed that amlodipine besylate–benazepril hydrochloride combination therapy is superior to monotherapy with either component drug in older patients with stage 2 hypertension, and is well tolerated [24].

Patients in the SELECT study were divided into those with isolated systolic hypertension (ISH; mean daytime systolic/diastolic blood pressure ≥150/<90 mmHg), and those with predominantly systolic hypertension (PSH; mean daytime systolic/diastolic blood pressure ≥150/90–100 mmHg) and the effects of treatment were compared in these two populations [26]. The efficacy results are shown in Figure 5.11 and demonstrate that amlodipine besylate–benazepril hydrochloride combination therapy was very effective in patients with ISH or PSH, and was more effective than either component drug as monotherapy. The side-effect profile was similar in all three treatment groups. Edema was less common in the combination therapy group (7.8%) than in the amlodipine besylate group (13.6%). Notably, patients with ISH tended to be more difficult to treat than those with PSH.

Effects of amlodipine besylate–benazepril hydrochloride treatment on patients with isolated systolic hypertension and predominantly systolic hypertension

	Predominantly systolic hypertension			Isolated systolic hypertension		
	A–B	A	B	A–B	A	B
N	76	63	78	53†	63	54
Mean 24h SBP	−21.1*	−14.0	−12.1	−19.6†	−11.7	−9.3
Mean 24h PP	−10.0*	−7.2	−5.7	−11.0†	−7.0	−5.0
Mean 24h DBP	−11.0*	−6.7	−6.4	−8.6	−4.7	−4.3
RR (%)	75.0*	47.6	37.2	71.7†	33.3	35.2
CR	63.2*	34.9	33.2	64.2†	23.8	29.6

*P<0.001 A/B compared with A and B; †P<0.001 A/B compared with A and B.

Figure 5.11 **Effects of amlodipine besylate–benazepril hydrochloride treatment on patients with isolated systolic hypertension and predominantly systolic hypertension.** A, amlodipine besylate; B, benazepril hydrochloride; CR, control rate; DBP, diastolic blood pressure; PP, pulse pressure; RR, relative risk; SBP, systolic blood pressure. Reproduced with permission from Neutel JM, Smith DHG, Weber MA, Nwose OM, Schofield L, Gatlin M. P-411. Management of isolated vs. predominantly systolic hypertension: results of the Systolic Evaluation of Lotrel Efficacy and Comparative Therapies (SELECT) study. Am J Hypertens 2004; 17 (5 Pt 2): 184A.

Open-label study comparing fosinopril monotherapy and amlodipine monotherapy, with fosinopril–amlodipine combination therapy used to achieve blood pressure control (FACET trial)

The primary aim of the Fosinopril versus Amlodipine Cardiovascular Events Randomized Trial (FACET) was to compare the effects of the ACE inhibitor fosinopril and the calcium channel blocker amlodipine on serum lipids and diabetes control in patients with hypertension and type 2 diabetes [27,28]. Prospectively defined cardiovascular events were assessed as secondary outcomes. A total of 380 patients with hypertension and type 2 diabetes were included in the study: 189 patients were randomly assigned to open-label fosinopril (20 mg/day) and 191 patients to amlodipine (10 mg/day) and followed for up to 3.5 years. If blood pressure was not controlled on the assigned study drug, the other study drug was added.

The results of the study showed that both treatments were effective in lowering blood pressure. Systolic blood pressure was significantly lower in the amlodipine group compared with the fosinopril group at the last visit (4 mmHg; P<0.01). There was no significant difference between the two groups in total serum cholesterol, HDL cholesterol, HbA1c, fasting serum glucose, or plasma insulin at the end of follow-up. The risk of the combined outcome of acute myocardial infarction, stroke, or hospitalized angina, however, was significantly lower in the patients who received fosinopril compared with those who received amlodipine (14/189 vs. 27/191; hazard ratio = 0.49, 95% CI = 0.26–0.95). Therefore, although fosinopril and amlodipine had similar effects on biochemical measures, and amlodipine caused a greater reduction than fosinopril in systolic blood pressure, the patients randomized to fosinopril had a significantly lower risk of major vascular events compared with the patients randomized to amlodipine.

To achieve blood pressure control, amlodipine was added for 58 of the 189 patients (30.7%) in the fosinopril group, and fosinopril was added in 50 of the 191 patients in the amlodipine group (26.2%). In the intention-to-treat analysis, the risk of cardiovascular events was not significantly different in patients who received the combination of fosinopril and amlodipine from those who received fosinopril alone, and both groups had a significantly lower cardiovascular risk than those who took amlodipine alone [29]. However, clinical outcome data on combination therapies with ACE inhibitors and calcium channel blockers in hypertension are inconclusive, and although extrapolations about efficacy of combination therapies based on FACET have been made by some authors [30], these are considered by others to be unwarranted [19].

Studies assessing angiotensin II receptor blockers in combination with calcium channel blockers

Fixed-dose combinations of an ARB (olmesartan or valsartan) with a calcium channel blocker (amlodipine) have recently been approved by the FDA. Olmesartan–amlodipine and valsartan–amlodipine fixed-dose combination therapies are very effective in treating hypertension and are well tolerated [31–38]. As well as effectively reducing blood pressure, these new fixed-dose combinations have been associated with significant reductions in the incidence of peripheral edema compared with amlodipine monotherapy [31,34,35], thus making them more acceptable to patients. Furthermore, the metabolic neutrality of the component drugs in these fixed-dose combination therapies may render them the preferred choice for the treatment of hypertensive patients with diabetes or the metabolic syndrome.

This section describes key studies that have been conducted to assess the efficacy and safety of olmesartan–amlodipine and valsartan–amlodipine combination therapies.

Double-blind, placebo-controlled study comparing olmesartan–amlodipine combination therapy with olmesartan and amlodipine monotherapies

A multicenter, randomized, double-blind, placebo-controlled factorial study was conducted to compare the efficacy and tolerability of olmesartan–amlodipine combination therapy with those of the component monotherapies in patients with mild to severe hypertension [39]. Eligible patients were naïve to antihypertensive therapy or had undergone a washout of previous antihypertensive therapy for up to 2 weeks, and had a seated diastolic blood pressure of 95–120 mmHg. A total of 1940 eligible patients were randomized to receive one of the following treatments for 8 weeks: olmesartan 10, 20 or 40 mg; amlodipine 5 or 10 mg; each possible combination of olmesartan and amlodipine; or placebo. The primary endpoint was the change from baseline in seated diastolic blood pressure at week 8. The mean blood pressure at baseline was 164/102 mmHg, and 79.3% of patients had stage 2 hypertension.

Olmesartan–amlodipine combination therapy was associated with dose-dependent reductions in seated diastolic blood pressure (from –13.8 mmHg with olmesartan 10 mg–amlodipine 5 mg to –19.0 mmHg with olmesartan 40 mg–amlodipine 10 mg) and seated systolic blood pressure (from –23.6 mmHg with olmesartan 20 mg–amlodipine 5 mg to –30.1 mmHg with olmesartan 40 mg–amlodipine 10 mg). These reductions were significantly greater than the reductions with the corresponding component monotherapies ($P < 0.001$; see Figure 5.12).

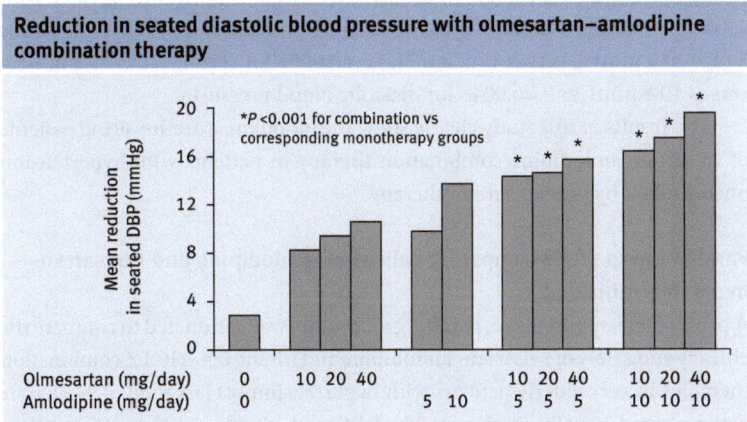

Reduction in seated diastolic blood pressure with olmesartan–amlodipine combination therapy

*P <0.001 for combination vs corresponding monotherapy groups

Figure 5.12 Reduction in seated diastolic blood pressure with olmesartan–amlodipine combination therapy. Data from [39].

At week 8, the percentage of patients who achieved the blood pressure goal (<140/90 mmHg; <130/80 mmHg for patients with diabetes) was 35.0–53.2% in the combination therapy groups, 20.0–36.3% in the olmesartan monotherapy groups, and 21.1–32.5% in the amlodipine monotherapy groups (P <0.005 combination therapies versus component monotherapies), compared with 8.8% in the placebo group.

In this study, olmesartan–amlodipine combination therapy was effective at reducing blood pressure and was well tolerated in patients with mild to severe hypertension.

Double-blind study assessing the efficacy of valsartan–amlodipine in patients with hypertension uncontrolled with previous monotherapy (EX-FAST study)

A randomized, double-blind, multicenter study was conducted to assess the efficacy of valsartan–amlodipine combination therapy in patients whose blood pressure remained uncontrolled with previous monotherapy (Exforge in Failure after Single Therapy [EX-FAST] study) [40]. Eligible patients were switched directly from monotherapy to valsartan 160 mg–amlodipine 5 mg (n=443) or valsartan 160 mg–amlodipine 10 mg (n=451).

After 16 weeks, blood pressure control (defined as <140/90 mmHg, with <130/80 mmHg for diabetics) was achieved in 72.7% of patients who received valsartan 160 mg–amlodipine 5 mg and in 74.8% of those who received valsartan 160 mg–amlodipine 10 mg. Incremental reductions from baseline in mean sitting systolic and diastolic blood pressures were significantly greater with valsartan 160 mg–amlodipine 10 mg than with valsartan 160 mg–amlodipine 5 mg (20.0 mmHg versus 17.5 mmHg; P =0.0003 for systolic, and 11.6 mmHg versus 10.4 mmHg; P =0.0046 for diastolic blood pressure).

The results of this study clearly show the blood pressure-lowering benefits of valsartan–amlodipine combination therapy in patients with hypertension uncontrolled by previous monotherapy.

Parallel group study comparing valsartan–amlodipine and irbesartan–hydrochlorothiazide

A prospective, randomized, parallel group study was conducted to compare the efficacy and safety of valsartan–amlodipine and irbesartan–HCTZ combination therapies in very elderly patients with hypertension [41]. A total of 94 eligible patients, aged 75 to 89 years, completed a 4-week placebo period and were then randomized to receive either valsartan 160 mg–amlodipine 5 mg or irbesartan

300 mg–HCTZ 12.5 mg for 24 weeks. Amlodipine or HCTZ doses were doubled after 4 weeks of active treatment in non-responders.

Ambulatory blood pressure was significantly reduced with both treatment combinations. The mean reductions in 24-hour, daytime and night-time ambulatory systolic/diastolic blood pressure for the valsartan–amlodipine group (−29.9/−15.6 mmHg; −28.6/−14.5 mmHg; −26.2/−17.4 mmHg, respectively) were similar to those in the irbesartan–HCTZ group (−29.6/−15.4 mmHg; −29.3/−14.9 mmHg; −25.4/−16.9 mmHg, respectively). Both combinations also significantly reduced clinical sitting and lying blood pressures, with no difference between treatments. Blood pressure changes from lying to standing position were significantly greater in the irbesartan–HCTZ group (−17.2/−9.1 mmHg) compared with the valsartan–amlodipine group (−10.1/−1.9 mmHg) (P <0.05 for systolic blood pressure and P <0.01 for diastolic blood pressure). Potassium was significantly decreased and uric acid significantly increased in the irbesartan–HCTZ group only.

In this study, the effectiveness of valsartan–amlodipine combination therapy was similar to that of irbesartan–HCTZ combination therapy in reducing ambulatory and clinical blood pressure in very elderly hypertensives; however, valsartan–amlodipine offered some advantages in terms of less pronounced orthostatic blood pressure changes and absence of metabolic adverse effects.

References

1. Chobanian AV, Bakris GL, Black HR, et al., Joint National Committee on Prevention, Detection, Evaluation, and Treatment of High Blood Pressure. National Heart, Lung, and Blood Institute; National High Blood Pressure Education Program Coordinating Committee. The seventh report of the Joint National Committee on Prevention, Detection, Evaluation, and Treatment of High Blood Pressure. Hypertension 2003; 42:1206–52.

2. Guidelines Committee: 2003 European Society of Hypertension. European Society of Cardiology guidelines for the management of arterial hypertension. J Hypertens 2003; 21:1011–53.

3. Unger T, McInnes GT, Neutel JM, Böhm M. The role of olmesartan medoxomil in the management of hypertension. Drugs 2004; 64(24):2731–9.

4. Bloom BS. Continuation of initial antihypertensive medication after 1 year of therapy. Clin Ther 1998; 20:671–81.

5. Neutel JM, Saunders E, Bakris GL, et al., INCLUSIVE Investigators. The efficacy and safety of low- and high-dose fixed combinations of irbesartan/hydrochlorothiazide in patients with uncontrolled systolic blood pressure on monotherapy: the INCLUSIVE trial. J Clin Hypertens 2005; 7(10):578–86.

6. Sowers JR, Neutel JM, Saunders E, et al., INCLUSIVE Investigators. Antihypertensive efficacy of irbesartan/HCTZ in men and women with the metabolic syndrome and type 2 diabetes. J Clin Hypertens 2006; 8(7):470–80.

7. Ofili EO, Ferdinand KC, Saunders E, et al. Irbesartan/HCTZ fixed combinations in patients of different racial/ethnic groups with uncontrolled systolic blood pressure on monotherapy. J Natl Med Assoc 2006; 98(4):618–26.

8. Neutel JM, Franklin SS, Oparil S, Bhaumik A, Ptaszynska A, Lapuerta P. Efficacy and safety of irbesartan/HCTZ combination therapy as initial treatment for rapid control of severe hypertension. J Clin Hypertens 2006; 8(12):850–7; quiz 858–9.

9. Neutel JM, Franklin SS, Lapuerta P, Bhaumik A, Ptaszynska A. A comparison of the efficacy and safety of irbesartan/HCTZ combination therapy with irbesartan and HCTZ monotherapy in the treatment of moderate hypertension. J Hum Hypertens 2008; 22:266–74.

10. Neutel JM, Klein C, Meinicke TW, Schumacher H. Long-term efficacy and tolerability of telmisartan as monotherapy and in combination with other antihypertensive medications. Blood Press 2002; 11(5):302–9.

11. White WB, Weber MA, Davidai G, Neutel JM, Bakris GL, Giles T. Ambulatory blood pressure monitoring in the primary care setting: assessment of therapy on the circadian variation of blood pressure from the MICCAT-2 Trial. Blood Press Monit 2005; 10(3):157–63.

12. Lacourcière Y, Poirier L, Lefebvre J. Expedited blood pressure control with initial angiotensin II antagonist/diuretic therapy compared with stepped-care therapy in patients with ambulatory systolic hypertension. Can J Cardiol 2007; 23(5):377–82.

13. Neutel JM, Smith DH, Weber MA, Wang AC, Masonson HN. Use of an olmesartan medoxomil-based treatment algorithm for hypertension control. J Clin Hypertens 2004; 6(4):168–74.

14. Izzo JL, Neutel JM, Silfani T, Dubiel R, Walker F. Efficacy and safety of treating stage 2 systolic hypertension with olmesartan and olmesartan/HCTZ: results of an open-label titration study. J Clin Hypertens 2007; 9(1):36–44.

15. Izzo JL, Neutel JM, Silfani T, Dubiel R, Walker F. Titration of HCTZ to 50 mg daily in individuals with stage 2 systolic hypertension pretreated with an angiotensin receptor blocker. J Clin Hypertens 2007; 9(1):45–8.

16. Izzo J, Neutel J, Dubiel R, Walker F. Metabolic effects and safety of hydrochlorothiazide (HCTZ) in combination with olmesartan medoxomil (OLM) in stage 2 systolic hypertension (HTN). Am J Hypertens 2005; 18 (5 Pt 2):64A. Posters: Antihypertensive drugs and pharmacology. P-159.

17. Ruoff G. ACE inhibitors and diuretics. The benefits of combined therapy for hypertension. Postgrad Med 1989; 85(3):127–32, 137–9.

18. Mourad JJ, Waeber B, Zannad F, Laville M, Duru G, Andréjak M; investigators of the STRATHE trial. Comparison of different therapeutic strategies in hypertension: a low-dose combination of perindopril/indapamide versus a sequential monotherapy or a stepped-care approach. J Hypertens 2004; 22(12):2379–86.

19. PROGRESS Collaborative Group. Effects of a perindopril-based blood pressure lowering regimen on cardiac outcomes among patients with cerebrovascular disease. Eur Heart J 2003; 24:475–84.

20. Chapman N, Huxley R, Anderson C, et al; Writing Committee for the PROGRESS Collaborative Group. Effects of a perindopril-based blood pressure-lowering regimen on the risk of recurrent stroke according to stroke subtype and medical history: the PROGRESS Trial. Stroke 2004; 35:116–21. Epub 2003 Dec 11.

21. Morisco C, Lembo G, Sarno D, et al. Benefits of combination therapy in hypertensive patients with associated coronary artery disease: a subgroup with specific demands. J Cardiovasc Pharmacol 1998; 31(Suppl 2):S27–33.

22. Messerli FH, Weir MR, Neutel JM. Combination therapy of amlodipine/benazepril versus monotherapy of amlodipine in a practice-based setting. Am J Hypertens 2002; 15(6):550–6.

23. Neutel JM, Smith DH, Weber MA. Effect of antihypertensive monotherapy and combination therapy on arterial distensibility and left ventricular mass. Am J Hypertens 2004; 17(1):37–42.

24. Neutel JM, Smith DH, Weber MA, Schofield L, Purkayastha D, Gatlin M. Efficacy of combination therapy with amlodipine besylate/benazepril hydrochloride for lowering systolic blood pressure in stage 2 hypertension. Am J Geriatr Cardiol 2006; 15(3):142–50.

25. Neutel JM, Smith DH, Weber MA, Schofield L, Purkayastha D, Gatlin M. Efficacy of combination therapy for systolic blood pressure in patients with severe systolic hypertension: the Systolic Evaluation of Lotrel Efficacy and Comparative Therapies (SELECT) study. J Clin Hypertens 2005; 7(11):641–6; quiz 647–8.

26. Neutel JM, Smith DH, Weber MA, Nwose OM, Schofield L, Gatlin M. Management of isolated vs. predominantly systolic hypertension: results of the systolic evaluation of Lotrel efficacy and comparative therapies (SELECT) study. Am J Hypertens 2004; 17:184A (poster P-411).

27. Tatti P, Pahor M, Byington RP, et al. Outcome results of the Fosinopril Versus Amlodipine Cardiovascular Events Randomized Trial (FACET) in patients with hypertension and NIDDM. Diabetes Care 1998; 21:597–603.

28. Califf RM, Granger CB. Hypertension and diabetes and the Fosinopril versus Amlodipine Cardiovascular Events Trial (FACET). More ammunition against surrogate end points. Diabetes Care 1998; 21:655–7.

29. Pahor M, Tatti P. The Fosinopril versus Amlodipine Cardiovascular Events Trial (FACET) and combination therapies. Am J Cardiol 1999; 83:819–20.

30. Sowers JR. Comorbidity of hypertension and diabetes: the fosinopril versus amlodipine cardiovascular events trial (FACET). Am J Cardiol 1998; 82(9B):15–19R.

31. Chrysant SG. Amlodipine/ARB fixed-dose combinations for the treatment of hypertension: focus on amlodipine/olmesartan combination. Drugs Today (Barc) 2008; 44(6):443–53.

32. Bakris GL. Combined therapy with a calcium channel blocker and an angiotensin II type 1 receptor blocker. J Clin Hypertens (Greenwich) 2008; 10(1 Suppl 1):27–32.

33. Brachmann J, Ansari A, Mahla G, Handrock R, Klebs S. Effective and safe reduction of blood pressure with the combination of amlodipine 5 mg and valsartan 160 mg in hypertensive patients not controlled by calcium channel blocker monotherapy. Adv Ther 2008; 25(5): 399–411.

34. Philipp T, Smith TR, Glazer R, et al. Two multicenter, 8-week, randomized, double-blind, placebo-controlled, parallel-group studies evaluating the efficacy and tolerability of amlodipine and valsartan in combination and as monotherapy in adult patients with mild to moderate essential hypertension. Clin Ther 2007; 29(4):563–80.

35. Plosker GL, Robinson DM. Amlodipine/valsartan: fixed-dose combination in hypertension. Drugs 2008; 68(3):373–81.

36. Krzesinski JM, Scheen AJ. [A first drug combination for the treatment of arterial hypertension with a calcium channel antagonist (amlodipine besylate) and an angiotensin receptor blocker (valsartan): Exforge.] [Article in French.] Rev Med Liege 2007; 62(11):688–94.

37. Smith TR, Philipp T, Vaisse B, et al. Amlodipine and valsartan combined and as monotherapy in stage 2, elderly, and black hypertensive patients: subgroup analyses of 2 randomized, placebo-controlled studies. J Clin Hypertens (Greenwich) 2007; 9(5):355–64.

38. Poldermans D, Glazes R, Kargiannis S, et al. Tolerability and blood pressure-lowering efficacy of the combination of amlodipine plus valsartan compared with lisinopril plus hydrochlorothiazide in adult patients with stage 2 hypertension. Clin Ther 2007; 29(2):279–89.

39. Chrysant SG, Melino M, Karki S, Lee J, Heyrman R. The combination of olmesartan medoxomil and amlodipine besylate in controlling high blood pressure: COACH, a randomized, double-blind, placebo-controlled, 8-week factorial efficacy and safety study. Clin Ther 2008; 30(4):587–604.

40. Allemann Y, Fraile B, Lambert M, Barbier M, Ferber P, Izzo JL Jr. Efficacy of the combination of amlodipine and valsartan in patients with hypertension uncontrolled with previous monotherapy: the Exforge in Failure after Single Therapy (EX-FAST) study. J Clin Hypertens (Greenwich) 2008; 10(3):185–94.

41. Fogari R, Zoppi A, Mugellini A, et al. Efficacy and safety of two treatment combinations of hypertension in very elderly patients. Arch Gerontol Geriatr. Epub ahead of print 2008 May 3.

Chapter 6

Combination therapy as first-line treatment

Lowering of the blood pressure limit that represents adequate control of hypertension from 140/90 mmHg to 130/85 mmHg (see Chapter 1) has inevitably worsened the recorded rates of control among hypertensive patients: patients who were considered controlled at 140/90 mmHg are no longer considered controlled, so the percentage of controlled patients has decreased. Also, significantly, the lower target for blood pressure has created a greater challenge for physicians, who were already having difficulty achieving the 140/90 mmHg goal in their patients. Many physicians are becoming despondent as they believe that the lower blood pressure goals are impossible to achieve in the majority of their patients. Indeed, the universally accepted blood pressure that is considered to represent adequate control of hypertension in medical practice continues to be 140/90 mmHg for all patients, apart from those with diabetes or renal disease, in whom a lower target of 130/80 mmHg is considered appropriate [1]: 140/90 mmHg is the recommendation for coronary artery disease in the seventh report of the Joint National Committee on Prevention, Detection, Evaluation, and Treatment of High Blood Pressure, but AHA recommends 130/80 mmHg for diabetics. New approaches to the treatment of hypertension are required to meet the challenges raised by the lower recommended blood pressure target.

There are many obstacles for the patient and the physician along the path between diagnosis of hypertension and achievement of blood pressure control. Figure 6.1 shows the complexity of management of hypertension and the challenges facing physicians as they attempt to improve blood pressure control in their patients [2]. The longer the period for which blood pressure control is attempted, the greater the number of obstacles, and the less likely it is that control will be achieved. Achieving blood pressure control earlier in the course of therapy may eliminate many potential obstacles and increase the likelihood of long-term blood pressure control.

J. M. Neutel, *Combination Therapy in Hypertension*,
DOI: 10.1007/978-1-908517-28-9_6, © Springer Healthcare 2011

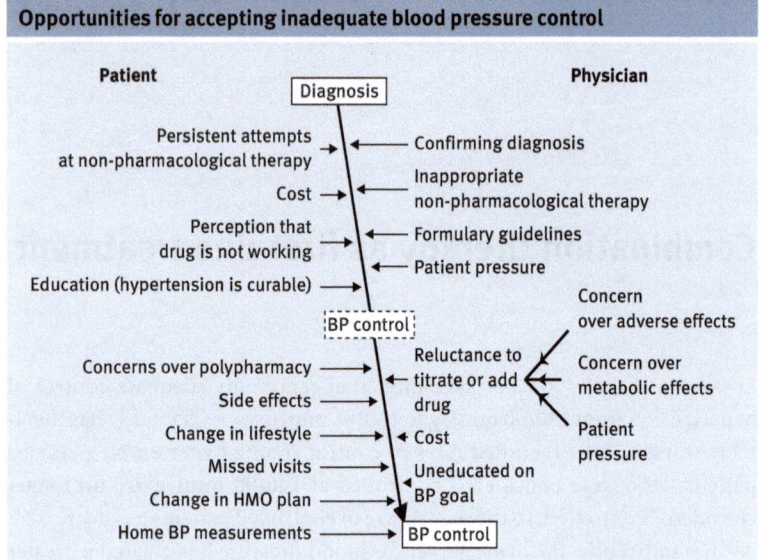

Figure 6.1 Opportunities for accepting inadequate blood pressure control. BP, blood pressure; HMO, health management organization. Reproduced with permission from Neutel JM, Smith DH, Weber MA. Low-dose combination therapy: an important first-line treatment in the management of hypertension. Am J Hypertens 2001; 14(3):286–92.

Use of low-dose combinations as first-line treatment

The best chance of controlling hypertension is with the initial treatment. A more aggressive approach to first-line treatment, achieving blood pressure control with the first dose, or the first few doses, of medication may significantly improve long-term control of blood pressure and decrease the acceptance of inadequate blood pressure control. Furthermore, changes in the approach to early management of hypertension are imperative to ensure significant reductions in the incidence of coronary artery disease in hypertensive patients. The earlier use of low-dose combination therapy in the management of hypertension may help significantly more patients achieve blood pressure control. The use of low-dose combination antihypertensive agents for first-line therapy will enable patients to take advantage of the cardiovascular benefits and blood pressure control that these agents provide early in the course of therapy [3]. Patients whose blood pressure is controlled rapidly after the initiation of antihypertensive therapy are convinced of the efficacy and necessity of their treatment and, therefore, are more likely to be compliant with medication. Initiating treatment of hypertensive patients with low-dose combination therapy may greatly improve rates of blood pressure control and reduce the incidence of coronary artery disease in treated hypertensive patients.

The seventh report of the Joint National Committee on Prevention, Detection, Evaluation, and Treatment of High Blood Pressure stresses the importance of reducing systolic blood pressure and notes that most patients will require at least two antihypertensive agents to achieve appropriate blood pressure goals [4]. The initial use of combination therapy is recommended in patients with stage 2 hypertension or with blood pressure more than 20/10 mmHg above the goal [4]. Highly effective combination therapies are needed to achieve more rigorous blood pressure control as recommended by the Joint National Committee and the World Health Organization.

Physicians have been reluctant to prescribe combination therapy as first-line treatment because they have believed that monotherapy is more convenient, less expensive and associated with fewer side effects than combination therapy, and that identifying which agent has caused an adverse event would be much more difficult with combination therapy than with mono-therapy [5]. As discussed in Chapter 3, all of these arguments can be refuted and, therefore, should not prevent the use of low-dose combination therapy as first-line treatment. Although physicians have for many years regarded the use of combination therapy as a last resort in the management of hypertension, typically limiting the use of combination treatment to 'problematic' patients later in therapy, there are numerous reasons why low-dose combination therapy may be excellent as a first-line treatment, or for use much earlier in the course of treating hypertension [6].

The advantages of low-dose combination therapy in the treatment of hyper-tension are shown in Figure 6.2. They are similar to the properties suggested for the ideal antihypertensive drug in Figure 3.1. Most importantly, first-line treatment with low-dose combination therapy may enable hypertensive patients to achieve better and earlier blood pressure control, with fewer adverse events, which may lead to improved patient compliance.

Low-dose combination drugs that are currently available for the treat-ment of hypertension are shown in Figure 6.3. To receive regulatory approval for initial therapy, low-dose combination agents are required to have greater efficacy and a more favorable adverse effect profile than each of their component drugs as monotherapy at the highest recommended dose. The only low-dose combination agents that have been given first-line approval by the United States' Food and Drug Administration are bisoprolol–hydrochlorothiazide (HCTZ), captopril–HCTZ, irbesartan–HCTZ (which has received a US license for first-line use in patients who are likely to require multiple drug therapy to achieve blood

Advantages of low-dose combination therapy in hypertension

- Effectively reduces blood pressure: greater efficacy than monotherapy because of the additive effect of complementary drugs on blood pressure and through neutralization of compensatory counter-regulatory reactions

- Provides 24-hour efficacy with once-a-day dosing as most of the low-dose combination drugs include long-acting components

- Higher response rate than monotherapy

- Effective in most subgroups of hypertensive patients because of the complementary nature of combination therapy

- Fewer, and less severe, dose-dependent adverse effects than monotherapy as blood pressure control is obtained at lower doses of each of the component drugs

- Fewer adverse metabolic effects than higher-dose monotherapy because these effects tend to be dose dependent

- End-organ protection beyond blood pressure control

- At least as convenient as monotherapy (once-a-day dosing and one dosage unit)

- Simplified titration

- Lower cost than monotherapy because low-dose combination therapy tends to be a little more expensive than each of the components but cheaper than if each of the components were used separately

- Improved therapeutic compliance

Figure 6.2 Advantages of low-dose combination therapy in hypertension.

pressure goals), valsartan–amlodipine and valsartan–HCTZ. Losartan–HCTZ has a limited first-line indication: this combination therapy is not indicated for initial therapy of hypertension, except when the hypertension is severe enough that the value of achieving prompt blood pressure control exceeds the risk of initiating combination therapy in these patients [7]. Other available combination agents have been given a second-line indication because they have a side-effect profile similar to one of their component agents. For example, low-dose angiotensin-converting enzyme (ACE) inhibitor–calcium-channel blocker combinations are more efficacious then either component drug alone, but they do not have a better adverse effect profile than ACE inhibitors as monotherapy because drug-related cough with ACE inhibitors is independent of dose; these combinations, therefore, do not qualify for first-line approval [6].

Fixed-dose combinations

Fixed-dose drug combinations for the treatment of hypertension have become increasingly popular in recent years. As discussed in Chapter 2, the rationale behind fixed-dose combination therapy is based on dose-dependent treatment benefits, where higher drug doses produce better hypertension control without an increase in adverse effects, provided the two drugs have complementary

Low-dose combination drugs for hypertension

Generic name	Brand name	Combination
ACE inhibitors		
Benazepril–amlodipine	Lotrel	ACE inhibitor + CCB
Benazepril–HCTZ	Lotensin HCT	ACE inhibitor + HCTZ
Captopril–HCTZ[a]	Capozide	ACE inhibitor + HCTZ
Enalapril–HCTZ	Vaseretic	ACE inhibitor + HCTZ
Lisinopril–HCTZ	Prinzide	ACE inhibitor + HCTZ
	Zestoretic	ACE inhibitor + HCTZ
Moexipril–HCTZ	Uniretic	ACE inhibitor + HCTZ
Monopril–HCTZ	Monopril HCT	ACE inhibitor + HCTZ
Perindopril–indapamide[b]	Preterax	ACE inhibitor + diuretic
Quinapril–HCTZ	Accuretic	ACE inhibitor + HCTZ
Trandolapril–verapamil	Tarka	ACE inhibitor + CCB
Angiotensin receptor blockers		
Candesartan–HCTZ	Atacand HCT	ARB + HCTZ
Irbesartan–HCTZ[a]	Avalide	ARB + HCTZ
	CoAprovel	ARB + HCTZ
Losartan–HCTZ[c]	Hyzaar	ARB + HCTZ
	Cozaar-Comp	ARB + HCTZ
Olmesartan– HCTZ	Benicar HCT	ARB + HCTZ
	Olmetic Plus	ARB + HCTZ
Telmisartan–HCTZ	Micardis HCT	ARB + HCTZ
Valsartan–HCTZ[a]	Diovan HCT	ARB + HCTZ
Olmesartan–amlodipine	Azor	ARB + CCB
Valsartan–amlodipine[a]	Exforge	ARB + CCB
β Blocker		
Bisoprolol–HCTZ[a,b]	Ziac	β blocker + HCTZ
Metoprolol–HCTZ	Lopressor HCT	β blocker + HCTZ
Renin inhibitor		
Aliskerin–HCTZ	Tekturna	Renin inhibitor + HCTZ

[a] Approved for first-line treatment in the USA.
[b] Approved for first-line treatment in the UK.
[c] Limited first-line indication in the USA.

Figure 6.3 Low-dose combination drugs for hypertension. Note: both brand names and availability vary from country to country. ACE, Angiotensin-converting enzyme; ARB, angiotensin II receptor blocker; CCB, calcium channel blocker; HCTZ, hydrochlorothiazide.

side effects. For example, a potassium-sparing drug, such as an ARB, can be combined with a potassium-losing drug, such as HCTZ.

Three recent studies highlight the benefits of fixed-dose combination therapy compared with monotherapy in the treatment of hypertension. In a large practice-based clinical study, fixed-dose combination therapy with amlodipine 5 mg–benazepril 10 mg or amlodipine 5 mg–benazepril 20 mg was shown to be safe and effective in the treatment of patients with mild-to-moderate hypertension who were either uncontrolled on, or intolerant of, amlodipine 5 mg or 10 mg monotherapy [8]. The amlodipine–benazepril combination was also associated with improved edema within 4 weeks of treatment in patients who presented with edema while on amlodipine monotherapy [8]. This study is discussed in Chapter 5 (pp. 56–58). In the SELECT study, amlodipine besylate 5 mg–benazepril hydrochloride 20 mg combination therapy was shown to be superior to monotherapy with either component drug in patients aged at least 55 years with stage 2 hypertension, and to be well tolerated [9–11]. This study is discussed in Chapter 5 (pp. 60–63). In a randomized, double-blind, parallel-group study, irbesartan 300 mg–HCTZ 25 mg combination therapy was shown to be associated with statistically significantly greater reductions in both systolic and diastolic blood pressures compared with either component as monotherapy in patients with moderate hypertension, and to be well tolerated [12]. This study is discussed in Chapter 5 (pp. 47–48).

References

1. Epstein M, Bakris G. Newer approaches to antihypertensive therapy. Use of fixed-dose combination therapy. Arch Intern Med 1996; 156:1969–78.
2. Neutel JM, Smith DH, Weber MA. Low-dose combination therapy: an important first-line treatment in the management of hypertension. Am J Hypertens 2001; 14(3):286–92.
3. Neutel JM. Low-dose antihypertensive combination therapy: its rationale and role in cardiovascular risk management. Am J Hypertens 1999;12:73S–79S.
4. The Seventh Report of the Joint National Committee on Prevention, Detection, Evaluation, and Treatment of High Blood Pressure. US Department of Health and Human Services. NIH Publication No. 04-5230. Bethesda, MD: National Institutes of Health, August 2004.
5. Neutel JM Combination therapy and the treatment of hypertension. Cardiology Special Edition 2003; 9(1 of 2):11–15.
6. Holzgreve H. Combination versus monotherapy as initial treatment in hypertension. Herz 2003; 28(8):725–32.
7. Food and Drug Administration, Center for Drug Evaluation and Research. Summary Minutes of the Cardiovascular and Renal Drugs Advisory Committee meeting on April 18, 2007. http://www.fda.gov/OHRMS/DOCKETS/AC/07/minutes/2007-4287m-minutes-final.pdf. Last accessed May 2011.
8. Messerli FH, Weir MR, Neutel JM. Combination therapy of amlodipine/benazepril versus monotherapy of amlodipine in a practice-based setting. Am J Hypertens 2002; 15:550–6.

9. Neutel JM, Smith DH, Weber MA, Schofield L, Purkayastha D, Gatlin M. Efficacy of combination therapy with amlodipine besylate/benazepril hydrochloride for lowering systolic blood pressure in stage 2 hypertension. Am J Geriatr Cardiol 2006; 15(3):142–50.

10. Neutel JM, Smith DH, Weber MA, Schofield L, Purkayastha D, Gatlin M. Efficacy of combination therapy for systolic blood pressure in patients with severe systolic hypertension: the Systolic Evaluation of Lotrel Efficacy and Comparative Therapies (SELECT) study. J Clin Hypertens 2005; 7(11):641–6; quiz 647–8.

11. Neutel JM, Smith DH, Weber MA, Nwose OM, Schofield L, Gatlin M. Management of isolated vs. predominantly systolic hypertension: results of the systolic evaluation of Lotrel efficacy and comparative therapies (SELECT) study. Am J Hypertens 2004; 17:184A (poster P-411).

12. Neutel JM, Franklin SS, Lapuerta P, Bhaumik A, Ptaszynska A. A comparison of the efficacy and safety of irbesartan/HCTZ combination therapy with irbesartan and HCTZ monotherapy in the treatment of moderate hypertension. J Hum Hypertens 2008; 22:266–74.

Chapter 7

Future combination agents

Possible combinations of first-line antihypertensive drugs are shown in Figure 7.1 [1]. Some combination therapies may prove to be particularly helpful in addressing coexisting morbidities as well as hypertension. For example, patients with hypertension and depressed cardiac function (congestive heart failure with decreased ejection fraction) may benefit from the combination of an angiotensin-converting enzyme (ACE) inhibitor and a diuretic. The combination of a calcium channel blocker and an ACE inhibitor may offer additional benefit to hypertensive patients with diabetes, although other combinations, such as an ACE inhibitor and a diuretic, may be used. Hypertensive patients with persist-

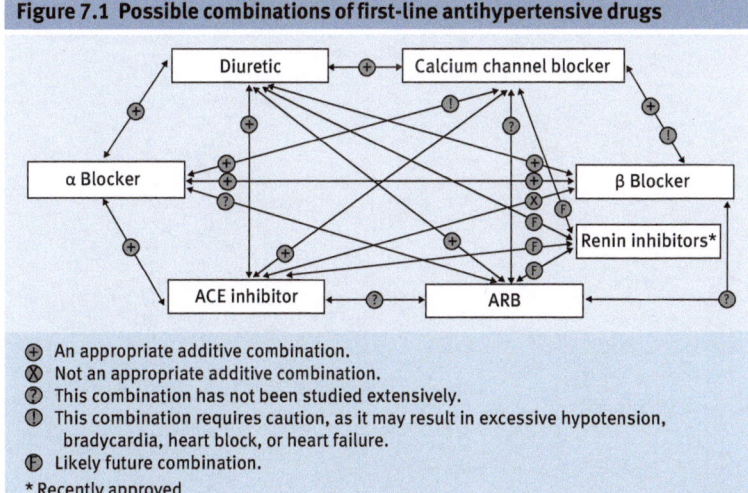

Figure 7.1 Possible combinations of first-line antihypertensive drugs

- ⊕ An appropriate additive combination.
- ⊗ Not an appropriate additive combination.
- ⑦ This combination has not been studied extensively.
- ① This combination requires caution, as it may result in excessive hypotension, bradycardia, heart block, or heart failure.
- Ⓕ Likely future combination.
- * Recently approved

Figure 7.1 Possible combinations of first-line antihypertensive drugs. ACE, angiotensin-converting enzyme; ARB, angiotensin II receptor blocker. Adapted with permission from Moser M, Prisant LM. Low-dose combination therapy in hypertension. Am Fam Physician 1997; 56:1275–6, 1279, 1282.

J. M. Neutel, *Combination Therapy in Hypertension*, 79
DOI: 10.1007/978-1-908517-28-9_7, © Springer Healthcare 2011

ent angina may respond well to treatment with a long-acting, dihydropyridine, calcium channel blocker combined with a β blocker; however, such a fixed-dose combination is not yet available.

Combination therapies that comprise four antihypertensive agents are being investigated [2].

A new class of drugs known as dual-acting receptor antagonists (DARA) may take the concept of combination therapy a step further. A DARA compound is a single molecule that combines two therapeutic modes of action. Clinical investigations are now underway for a DARA compound that blocks both angiotensin II and endothelin 1 receptors.

References

1. Neutel JM. Combination therapy and the treatment of hypertension. Cardiology Special Edition 2003; 9(1 of 2):11–15.
2. Mahmud A, Feely J. Low-dose quadruple antihypertensive combination: more efficacious than individual agents – a preliminary report. Hypertension 2007; 49(2):272–5.

Chapter 8

Clinical inertia in the management of hypertension

Complete control of blood pressure is rare in clinical practice, particularly in high-risk patients, and there are many opportunities for accepting inadequate hypertension control (see Figure 6.1). As mentioned in Chapter 1, patient-related factors clearly contribute to poor control of hypertension; however, physician-related factors, including 'passive' clinical inertia (also known as therapeutic inertia), are also partly responsible [1]. Clinical inertia, defined as the provider's failure to increase antihypertensive medications when blood pressure is ≥140/90 mmHg, has been suggested to be an important factor that contributes to suboptimal blood pressure control rates in hypertensive patients [2,3]. Clinical inertia derives from poorly prescribed lifestyle changes, excess reliance on monotherapy, and scarce on-treatment modifications [4].

Studies demonstrating impact of clinical inertia

In hypertension management, the effects of clinical inertia on blood pressure control have been assessed in a study that used data from over 12,000 uncontrolled hypertensive patients [2]. Blood pressure values and medication doses at each visit to the physician were analyzed and clinical inertia scores calculated. The second visit to the physician was designated the index visit (individuals had to have elevated blood pressure at this visit to qualify for the analysis), and the fourth visit was designated the outcome visit. Data from the second and third visits were used to calculate a clinical inertia score for each patient (score of 0 = no inertia; 1 = partial inertia; 2 = total inertia). A clinical inertia rate for each provider was also calculated (total number of changes in medications in visits with elevated blood pressure divided by total number of visits with elevated blood pressure) to give a rate between 0 (no inertia) and

J. M. Neutel, *Combination Therapy in Hypertension*,
DOI: 10.1007/978-1-908517-28-9_8, © Springer Healthcare 2011

1 (complete inertia). The data analysis showed that antihypertensive therapy was increased during 20% of visits by patients for whom blood pressure exceeded 140/90 mmHg. Furthermore, there was a statistically significantly greater decrease in systolic blood pressure in patients with no clinical inertia compared with those with total clinical inertia ($P \leq 0.0001$). Factors associated with a higher patient clinical inertia score included a higher provider clinical inertia rate ($P <0.005$), white patients ($P <0.03$), fewer medications at the index visit ($P \leq 0.0001$) and older age ($P \leq 0.0001$). Not surprisingly, patients with higher clinical inertia scores had lower rates of blood pressure control ($P <0.0001$). The results of the analysis also showed that the clinical inertia rate of providers predicted the clinical inertia score for their patients, and the clinical inertia score for patients predicted whether there was blood pressure control to less than 140/90 mmHg. This study confirms that clinical inertia in hypertension management is common and has a significant adverse effect on blood pressure control.

The impact of clinical inertia on blood pressure control in hypertensive patients has also been investigated in a retrospective cohort study of 7253 patients who had at least four hypertension-related physician visits and at least one elevated blood pressure in a 1-year period (see Figure 8.1) [3]. A 1-year clinical inertia score was calculated for each patient as the difference between expected and observed medication change rates, with higher scores reflecting greater clinical inertia. Antihypertensive therapy was increased during 13.1% of visits by patients with uncontrolled blood pressure. Systolic blood pressure decreased in patients in the lowest quintile of the clinical inertia score, but increased in those in the highest quintile (−6.8 mmHg versus +1.8 mmHg; $P <0.001$). Individuals in the lowest clinical inertia quintile were approximately 33 times more likely to have their blood pressure controlled at the last visit than those in highest quintile (odds ratio 32.7; 95% CI 25.1–42.6; $P <0.0001$). Clinical inertia accounted for around 19% of the variance in blood pressure control. If clinical inertia scores were decreased by around 50%, i.e. medication dosages were increased during around 30% of visits, blood pressure control would increase from the observed 45.1% to a projected 65.9% in 1 year. This study confirms the high rate of clinical inertia in uncontrolled hypertensive patients, and emphasizes the major impact that clinical inertia has on blood pressure control in hypertensive patients who are receiving regular care.

A further study of 800 hypertensive men (mean age 65.5 years) over a 2-year period showed that approximately 40% of the patients had a blood pressure of at least 160/90 mmHg despite an average of more than six hypertension-related

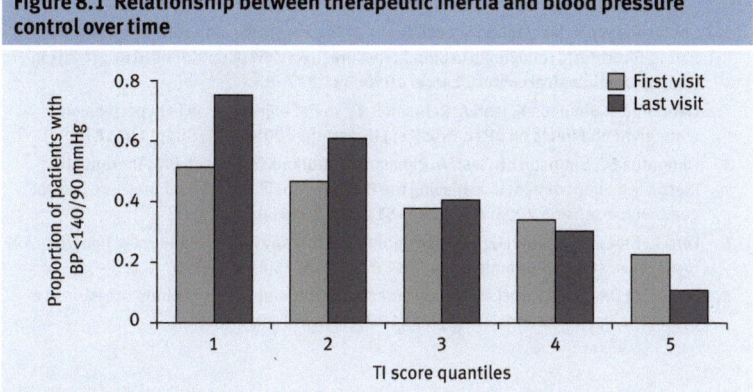

Figure 8.1 Relationship between therapeutic inertia and blood pressure control over time. Quintile 1 included patients who experienced the least TI, quintile 5 the most. For the trend $P < 0.001$. BP, blood pressure; TI, therapeutic inertia. Data from [3].

visits to the physician per year [5]. Increases in antihypertensive therapy occurred during 6.7% of visits and were associated with increased levels of both systolic and diastolic blood pressure at that visit (but not previous visits), a previous change in therapy, the presence of coronary artery disease, or a scheduled visit. Patients who had more intensive therapy had significantly better control of blood pressure ($P < 0.01$). During the 2-year period, systolic blood pressure decreased by 6.3 mmHg among patients with the most intensive treatment and increased by 4.8 mmHg among the patients with the least intensive treatment. The results of this study show that patients who received more intensive medical therapy had better blood pressure control.

Conclusions

Improving the treatment of hypertension requires an understanding of the ways in which physicians manage this condition and a means of assessing the efficacy of patient care [5]. The studies described above highlight physician inertia as an issue that may prevent many patients from achieving guideline-recommended blood pressure goals, and support the concept that many physicians are not aggressive enough in their approach to hypertension. A well-established blood pressure goal results in physicians being more aggressive in their management of blood pressure. Furthermore, a treat-to-target approach and combination therapy (which is always more effective than drug titration) can help the majority of patients reach blood pressure goals.

References

1. Collins R, Peto R, MacMahon S, et al. Blood pressure, stroke, and coronary heart disease. Part 2, Short-term reductions in blood pressure: overview of randomised drug trials in their epidemiological context. Lancet 1990; 335:827–38.

2. Okonofua E, Simpson K, Jesri A, Rehman S, Egan B. Clinical inertia in hypertension management: Effects on BP control. Am J Hypertens 2005; 18(5; Suppl 1):41A (P-93).

3. Okonofua EC, Simpson KN, Jesri A, Rehman SU, Durkalski VL, Egan BM. Therapeutic inertia is an impediment to achieving the Healthy People 2010 blood pressure control goals. Hypertension 2006; 47(3):345–51. Epub 2006 Jan 23.

4. Ferri C, Croce G, Desideri G. Role of combination therapy in the treatment of hypertension: focus on valsartan plus amlodipine. Adv Ther 2008; 25(4):300–320.

5. Berlowitz DR, Ash AS, Hickey EC, et al. Inadequate management of blood pressure in a hypertensive population. N Engl J Med 1998; 339(27):1957–63.